Pharmacy in Senegal

DONNA A. PATTERSON

Pharmacy in Senegal

Gender, Healing, and Entrepreneurship

INDIANA UNIVERSITY PRESS

Bloomington and Indianapolis

This book is a publication of

Indiana University Press
Office of Scholarly Publishing
Herman B Wells Library 350
1320 East 10th Street
Bloomington, Indiana 47405 USA

iupress.indiana.edu

Telephone   800-842-6796
Fax   812-855-7931

Manufactured in the United States of America

Library of Congress Cataloging-in-Publication Data

Patterson, Donna A., author.
    Pharmacy in Senegal : gender, healing, and entrepreneurship / Donna A. Patterson.
    p. ; cm.
    Includes bibliographical references and index.
    ISBN 978-0-253-01470-2 (cl : alk. paper) — ISBN 978-0-253-
01475-7 (pb : alk. paper) — ISBN 978-0-253-01478-8 (eb)
    I. Title.
    [DNLM: 1. Community Pharmacy Services—Senegal. 2. Pharmacies—Senegal.
3. Pharmacists—Senegal. 4. Women, Working—Senegal. QV 737 HS1]
    RA401.S4
    362.17'82009663—dc23

                                                                2014037488

1 2 3 4 5   20 19 18 17 16 15

*To the memory of my grandmother and my Aunt Josie,
from whom I draw inspiration.*

Contents

Acknowledgments

This book project has been a labor of love. I chose to write a history of Senegal's pharmacists because of the dearth of research on this topic and my profound interest in the subject matter. No one had ever written on the history of the pharmacy profession in Senegal; indeed, only two works (by Didier Fassin and Diane Barthel, an anthropologist and sociologist, respectively) had even considered this medical class. I knew that the undertaking would be daunting but I was eager to begin reconstructing this history. I thoroughly enjoyed this journey, and I am grateful to the scholars, colleagues, supporters, and informants on both sides of the Atlantic Ocean who have propelled me along the way.

Staff at the Archives nationales du Sénégal, the Archives d'Amicale Santé Navale et d'Outre Mer (ASNOM), and the Council for the Development of Social Science Research in Africa (CODESRIA), such as Mamadou N'diaye, Jean-François Le Blanc, and Jean-Pierre Diouf, have helped to facilitate the completion of this project. In addition, I am grateful for visits to the library at ENDA-Tiers Monde in Dakar, Senegal, and to the Centre des Archives d'Outre-Mer in Aix-en-Provence. These trips were funded through generous financial support from Fulbright IIE, Indiana University's Kelly School of Business and Department of History, the West African Research Association, the Woodrow Wilson Center, UNCF-Mellon, the Institute for the Medical Humanities at the University of Texas Medical Branch (UTMB), and Wellesley College.

In Senegal, in particular, I owe my deepest gratitude to pharmacists and other informants who shared their oral histories, published and unpublished documents, and photographs. In particular, I wish to thank Maïmouna Diop, N'deye Dieynaba Fall, N'deye Toutane Thiam Ngom, Majhemout Diop, and Rito Alcantara. Over the years, office holders and staff at the Ordre national des pharmaciens (National Order of Pharmacists) have been particularly supportive: Mamadou Ndiadé, Cheikhou Oumar Dia, Liliane Traoré, and Yasmine Tall. Others in Senegal also provided support: Charles Becker, Boubacar Barry, and Abdoulahat Mangane. Many thanks to the Council for the Development of Social Science Research in Africa (CODESRIA) and the West African Research Center (WARC) for providing academic affiliation at different stages of this project. In addition, several people and their families helped make my time in Senegal "a home away from home," especially Rougui Diaw, Youhanidou Wane, and the entire Gassama family. My warmest appreciation is extended to Awa Hyzagi, one of my best friends. Her siblings, mother, and extended family have made an indelible mark on my life.

Stateside, I owe enormous gratitude to people in a number of cities. John H. Hanson, the chair of my dissertation committee, was a chair-exemplar, who has successfully managed numerous dissertations in the 1990s and 2000s with quiet reserve and impeccable leadership. I had not yet met him when he agreed to become the chair of my graduate committee while he was on a sabbatical in Ghana. In the end, I could never have envisioned a better advisor. In addition to John's guidance, other faculty at Indiana University had a huge influence on my professional development: Eileen Julien, Phyllis Martin, Gracia Clark, and Peter Guardino. In Bloomington, too, a number of friends made life bearable, especially Candis Smith, Yerim Fall, Stephanie Shonekan, and Katy Fallon. While writing my dissertation, I worked at Dillard University in New Orleans. There I joined a cohort of junior faculty who were fierce collaborators on projects and pedagogy: Ras Michael Brown, Rhetta Seymour, and Uchenna Vasser. Marshall Stevenson, who was dean of social sciences at Dillard University, offered me my first full-time teaching job.

At Wellesley College, numerous colleagues on campus and at other institutions have offered support by reading a component of the project or engaging in conversation. At Wellesley College, I would like to thank Susan Reverby, Wilbur Rich, Eve Zimmerman, and my colleagues in the Africana Studies department. Africanist and African diaspora scholars from other institutions, such as Liz McMahon,

Jackie Woodfork, Joye Bowman, Ras Michael Brown, Kairn Kleiman, and Elias Bongmba, have offered encouragement and stimulating discussions. In addition to faculty, I owe gratitude to others: Brahima Ouattara, who provided research support in Dakar, and Sophie Merlin, who helped me to transcribe digital files in Wellesley. I wish to thank the anonymous reviewers of this manuscript for their generous comments. It was a pleasure working with Dee Mortensen, a sponsoring editor at Indiana University Press. From our first conversations about the premise of this work to the final stages of production, I could never have imagined that this process would be as enjoyable as it has been.

Several members of my family provided profound encouragement while I worked on the stages of this project. Special thanks go to my grandmother, my mother, my sister, and Sonya. Finally, my most heartfelt thanks go to Amadou and Leila for their patience while I travel the world and sometimes sequester myself in my home office.

Pharmacy in Senegal

Introduction

Whenever someone asks me for directions in Senegal, I often respond in relation to the closest pharmacy. Pharmacies are my point
of reference, the lens through which I naturally read Senegal. Situated throughout the greater Dakar metropolitan area, pharmacies
are found in neighborhoods of all socioeconomic strata. There are
more pharmacies per capita in Senegal than in most West African
countries. I had encountered many pharmacies during early trips
to Senegal in the 1990s. However, it was not until I was selecting a
dissertation topic on the North American side of the Atlantic that I
chose to highlight pharmacy owners. My dissertation was on women
who owned pharmacies. However, male voices loomed large during
subsequent trips, and I examine both male and female pharmacists
in this book.[1]

During the nascent stages of the project, I corresponded with
Madame Fall, *née* N'deye Dieynaba Mbodj, across the Atlantic. Her
daughter Rama, a practicing pharmacist in Connecticut, fielded my
questions and relayed her mother's answers back via phone and
e-mail. It was a coup to secure Madame Fall as an informant, virtually or otherwise. Madame Fall, who owns Pharmacie Nouvelle
in Pikine, had just resigned after twenty years as president of Senegal's National Order of Pharmacists. In fact, she was one of the most
powerful pharmacists not just in Senegal but in all of West Africa.
She thus offered a great entrée into medical professionalization and
entrepreneurship in Senegal. Her extensive reminiscences on the
postcolonial realities of the profession were particularly revealing.

A few months later, I learned that Madame Fall was visiting a
second daughter who was enrolled in a pharmacy program at Howard
University and that she was willing to meet with me in person in

Washington, D.C. It was a snowy day, and I left work early and took a series of buses over to meet her. Of course, she was as gracious and elegant as I had imagined her to be, and our meeting was productive. One of the key things she told me that day was that women owned at least 50 percent of the pharmacies in Dakar, the Senegalese capital. This was impressive, given women's unequal access to education. In the early phase of my research project, I set out to prove or disprove this kernel of information.

In fact, I learned that women did own a large percentage of pharmacies; in Dakar, the number was even higher than her estimate. By the end of the twentieth century, women owned 65 percent of the pharmacies in Dakar and about half—48 percent—of the pharmacies nationwide. This study has grown from a history of female pharmacists into a broader examination of the medical professionalization of both men and women in postcolonial Senegal.

This book is a history of the evolution of health care in Senegal, where pharmacists played a critical role in the expansion of health care delivery. In particular, I focus on the role of Senegalese pharmacists in the country's public health sector from 1919 to 2000. Prior to the region's colonization by the French, traditional healers were the primary source of health care. Through colonial expansion and exchange, the French brought new healing techniques, and they also spread global disease. In their efforts to promote health in the colony, French colonial medical officials sought to impart knowledge of European medical systems to the local population. Training Senegalese pharmacists was part of this effort. Serving as a history of pharmacy instruction, practice, and ownership in Senegal, this book investigates the emergence of African biomedical professionals in the early twentieth century, the expansion of the profession, and the rise of female pharmacists. It offers new perspectives on the history of medical professionals in Africa.

One of my arguments is that pharmacists are central to biomedical care in Senegal, especially in Dakar, where many pharmacists own their businesses and provide services that go far beyond the sale of medicine. In Senegal, pharmacists are more numerous and more accessible to the public than physicians. They are at the forefront of health care, and often find themselves examining, diagnosing, and prescribing for the sick and ailing who come to their shops. Pharmacists have proved themselves instrumental as biomedical cultural intermediaries by delivering both health care and medical knowledge to the general population from the early decades of the twentieth century to the present. This book is the first work to chart the historical transformations of Senegalese pharmaceutical practice over the twentieth century by examining pharmaceutical training, health care providers and entrepreneurs, and social and familial pressures.

My work draws on the life histories of pharmacists, both male and female, and contextualizes their careers in the history of formal education and health care in twentieth-century Senegal. Among them are Rito Alcantara and Majhemout Diop, who studied pharmacy in Bordeaux and Dakar, respectively, during the 1940s. Both men wrote accounts of their education and professional practice in Europe and Africa during the colonial period. Both also had global connections: Alcantara was a member of international organizations such as the Red Cross, and Diop was an African Marxist and opposition leader who spent many years in exile abroad. I interviewed each of them several times, gaining valuable insight into colonial and postcolonial pharmacy practice.

Several women pharmacists are also highlighted in this book. I pay particular attention to a core group of women who have transformed ideas about gender roles, professional practice, and leadership in this predominately Muslim country. They include Solange Decupper, N'deye Dieynaba Fall, and Khady Bao, who held early leadership roles in postcolonial Senegal. These women are the pioneers who, as symbols and sometimes as mentors, helped to challenge biases against female pharmacists. The prominent role of women in this predominately Muslim nation is unique in the region. Decupper, Fall, and Bao were followed by a younger generation of men and women like Pape N'diaye, Maïmouna Diop, N'deye Toutane Ngom, and Nafissatou Mbaye, who built on professional traditions and technological innovations to thrive in the globalized pharmaceutical market of the late twentieth century. Male and female pharmacists play a significant role in providing health care in local communities and in managing regional and global health initiatives. Although overlooked in previous studies of Francophone African and Senegalese medical history, these professionals are critical figures in the history of biomedical incorporation and expansion in the region.

In the postcolonial period, beginning in 1960, Senegal expanded upon the colonial development of biomedical training and infrastructure to become a model of biomedical care and intervention. Future medical professionals came from Francophone West, North, and Central Africa to train at Senegalese medical schools and biomedical facilities. As Senegalese medical care evolved, pharmacists became the core of the health care system, and their critical role afforded them special status in this developing nation.

The local health care industry, while a model in West Africa, is not without its imperfections. While several of Senegal's biomedical facilities are comparable to those found in developed economies, major disparities remain. In particular, rural areas have less access to health care than urban ones. Additionally, like most other sub-Saharan African countries, Senegal only manufactures a fraction (in its case, 15–20 percent) of the pharmaceuticals it uses. As a result, the country remains dependent on foreign countries for its drug supply, with most coming from France, followed by other Western European countries. In the last twenty years, it has begun to develop relationships with new pharmaceutical partners, especially Morocco, India, China, and the United States.

In addition to formal pharmaceutical networks, pharmacists must also navigate drug sales in Senegal's unregulated, informal pharmaceutical sector. Pharmacists also facilitate health initiatives by the Senegalese state, USAID, PEPFAR, Oxfam, and other NGOs and government organizations. Because Senegalese pharmacists are the most accessible biomedical health care providers, they are key intermediaries at both the local and global level and major factors in Senegal's health economy.

While scholars have examined the role of African women workers in many professions, and other studies have looked at the professionalization of African medical personnel, this study of the pharmaceutical field in Senegal suggests a paradigm shift in the interplay between gender and medical professional development. Previous research on African medical personnel has focused primarily on doctors, nurses, and midwives, and very little material has been written about pharmacists.[2] In fact, pharmacists in most of Africa are often discussed only as supporting actors on the stage of public health or women's professionalization, and are dismissed as minor participants in broad studies of medical professionals.[3] Only a few studies of South Africa highlight the practice of pharmacy. Similarly, though existing literature has examined the economic activity of African women employed in the informal as well as the formal sector, no studies to date have highlighted female medical professionals in previously male-dominated industries, and certainly none have focused on female African pharmacists.[4] In this book, I begin to address some of the silence by examining women's professional negotiations in the formal sectors of African economies. This study is significant not only because it is the first historical study of Senegalese pharmacists, but also because it challenges our understandings of women's economic activity. In sum, this work contributes to the history of medicine, colonial studies, and modern African history.

This book also expands upon earlier studies of medical professionalization and gender by looking more comprehensively at training and by examining both men's and women's access to traditionally white-collar professions. It offers new scholarly perspectives on the acquisition of property and considers the ways in which male and female pharmacists are perceived in their communities, and how they negotiate these perceptions. It thus responds to the rising demand for publications on health and for English-language studies of Francophone Africa.

Situating Senegal in Historical Context

Senegal is a part of the larger Muslim world; its population is 94 percent Muslim. Islam arrived early in the West African subregion and was dominant in the ruling communities of the precolonial states of Mali and Songhai. For centuries these states dominated local and regional politics, and they facilitated trade along long-established networks throughout much of the Sahel and sub-Saharan West Africa. Before being colonized by the French, Senegal also participated in various trade networks extending into the Sahara and the northern Atlantic, along which passed horses, cattle, salt, gold, and ironwork. In addition, religious rituals, ideas, scholars, and brotherhoods were reproduced and created in the communities traversed by these trans-Saharan and trans-Sahelian networks. The Senegalese largely converted to Islam in the eighteenth and nineteenth centuries, at the same time that European colonial officials, especially the French, were spreading throughout Senegal. By the end of the colonial period, 90 percent of Senegal's population practiced Islam. Senegal today is diverse, with both Muslim and Christian faiths and African, Arab, and European influences intersecting to create something distinctively Senegalese. The peaceful coexistence of the Muslim majority with the Christian minority is indicated by the fact that Senegal's first postcolonial president, elected in 1960 and serving until 1980, was Léopold Sédar Senghor, a Catholic. The pharmacists highlighted in this study evoke this diversity, as does the medical knowledge they dispense.

Medical knowledge and medicines were also exchanged along these transnational networks. Healers and merchants disseminated them in their homes, at markets, and through migration. In Senegal in particular, the Serer, the Haalpulaar, and the Wolof all had healing traditions. For example, Serer healers used spiritual and herbal remedies for different types of disease. In the Serer worldview, diseases were caused by *karanta* ("contagion"), *kadow* ("magical contagion," from an evil source), and *nimil* (a type of physical defect).[5] Medicines included tinctures, capsules, and teas, all made from local and imported plant products. The Wolof, along with the Lébou, also practiced a spiritual intercession called *n'döep* that often involves trance and multiple participants to treat mental illness.[6] The medical knowledge systems active in Senegal were connected to translocal approaches to health and healing.

The country of Senegal today, however, cannot be understood without examining its colonial background. The period from the early eighteenth century through the mid-nineteenth century was critical to the development of French colonial power in Africa. In 1817, France reestablished the coastal settlements in Senegal that it had initiated as part of its colonial empire in the seventeenth century. By 1848, Senegal had formally become a French colony. It formed the base from which the French expanded into the West African interior, especially in the late nineteenth century during what is known as the "Scramble for Africa," when numerous European powers seized territories. In the last two decades of the nineteenth century, the French established four communes in Senegal unlike any other cities in West African colonial history: Saint-Louis (1872), Gorée Island (1880), Rufisque (1880), and Dakar (1887). African inhabitants of these four communes had conditional access to education, wage labor, and politics. Most were classed as *originaires*, with limited access to colonial services, while those who met educational and social requirements could be considered *évolués* (evolved), with greater political and economic opportunities.

Senegal became one of France's most important colonies, with the headquarters of French West Africa (Afrique occidentale française, AOF) situated within its borders. As the regional seat of AOF, Senegal benefited from the significant development of infrastructure by the French, such as roads, railroads, medical facilities, schools, and administrative buildings. This investment in education and infrastructure would come to benefit African health care personnel in the twentieth century. Moreover, human resources were a key ingredient in France's colonial health policy. French nationals trained in medicine, pharmacy, and other medical fields were stationed in French West Africa and other French colonies. In the late nineteenth century, the French began training small numbers of Africans as auxiliary staff to support French medical professionals.

Global and local disease epidemics, the scarcity of French personnel, and economic losses from World War I all contributed to a greater push for the education of African medical personnel in the late nineteenth and early twentieth centuries. As France's colonial empire neared its apogee between 1870 and 1918, it encountered a number of political challenges, including the ramifications of a series of epidemics in its colonies. As France sought to reallocate its medical personnel to respond to crises in a variety of locations, existing resources were stretched thin, and French colonial officials recognized the need to train medical personnel in the colonies.

France thus reorganized its overseas medical facilities and personnel. In 1890, an overseas branch of the Pasteur Institute was opened in Hanoi.[7] The Hanoi branch was followed by others in Madagascar (1901), Congo (1910), and Senegal (1913).[8] Microbiology and chemistry labs, scientific missions, hospitals, and other facilities were established throughout the colonies during this period as well, and the 1912 report of the inspector of civil health services for the French colonial missions indicates that there were hopes of opening a school of medicine in French West Africa.[9] However, although colonial bureaucrats discussed the possibility in concrete terms, the outbreak of both bubonic plague and World War I in 1914 postponed the opening of the facility.

With the end of the war, colonial administrators were spurred to accelerate the training of African personnel, and the push for the school of medicine increased. In October 1916, a new section for the pursuit of medical studies was created on Gorée Island, and on 1 November 1918, the School of Medicine for French West Africa finally opened.[10] Between 1919 and 1930 new sections were added in Senegal as well as in Bamako, Mali, to train pharmacists (1919), midwives, nurses, and veterinarians.[11] This commitment to African medical training would lead to a new social class of African professionals.

Research and Methodology

The material for this book was largely gathered during archival and ethnographic research trips to Dakar, Paris, and Aix-en-Provence in 2000–2001, 2005, 2008, 2009, and 2011. In Senegal, the bulk of the research was done in Dakar with supplementary trips to other areas, including Guèdiwaye, Diourbel, Pikine, and Thiaroye. I collected archival research, made numerous observational trips, and examined meeting minutes and other private correspondence. I also conducted many in-depth, semistructured interviews in French, asking more than sixty people (pharmacists and others) about their education and professional development, and about the benefits and limits of pharmacy ownership. Most of the conversations were recorded and a two-page questionnaire was used to maintain the integrity of the interviews. The questions explored the social profile of pharmacists, the circumstances that led people to earn a degree in pharmacy, customers' perceptions of them, shifting attitudes toward health care, and the obstacles informants had faced and how they had surmounted them. I sometimes followed up on interesting responses, leading to other threads of inquiry. In addition to interviewing pharmacists, I visited traditional healing hospitals and met with healers in greater Dakar.[12]

All informants participated voluntarily. My primary goal was to obtain personal reminiscences of medical training, practice, and ownership, using these interviews to fill the silences in the social history of pharmacy practice. Most interviews with pharmacists were done in their pharmacies, while others were conducted in offices at the headquarters of the National Order of Pharmacists, in administrative offices, and in the homes of pharmacy owners. All interviews with healers employing traditional methods were conducted at their work sites. I interviewed them to gain a better understanding of some patients' simultaneous use of biomedical care and other forms of healing. These varied methodological approaches are combined to create the analytical trajectory of this history.

The extensive field research I conducted in Dakar helped me to reaffirm existing contacts with pharmacists and to greatly multiply my research participants. Strong support from N'deye Dieynaba Fall and Maïmouna Diop, two powerful female pharmacists in greater Dakar, helped garner support from other pharmacists. Dr. Diop mailed a letter introducing me to all female pharmacists in the metropolitan area, and gave me a copy to use in requesting interviews outside of the immediate region and with male pharmacists.[13] In addition to biomedical health care providers, I also interviewed traditional herbalists and some of those involved in the illicit pharmaceutical market. While I was not able to gain access to all the pharmacists I queried, I was able to interview a diverse group of pharmacists who were at different stages of their career and were located in different neighborhoods and communities. These geographical and professional variations helped produce a diverse research sample.

This book is divided into two parts. The two chapters that make up the first section chronicle the development of colonial biomedicine in Senegal and focus on the factors that promoted the development of African medical professionals, especially pharmacists, during the colonial period. The second section, consisting of three chapters, concerns how men and women negotiated pharmacy ownership, navigated social tensions, and responded to global phenomena. These chapters discuss a range of both private and professional issues shaping pharmacists' lives. Chapters 1 and 5 rely heavily on the colonial archive, and chapter 2 liberally incorporates material from archival records, oral interviews, and other primary sources. The methodology used in chapters 3 and 4 integrates oral interviews, government records, and material from postcolonial professional organizations.

Chapter 1 introduces and highlights the significance of the creation of a class of African medical professionals in French West Africa, by examining late nineteenth-century France and the country's relationship with its colonies. It also details the creation of the Jules Carde School of Medicine and Pharmacy in 1918 and the increase in the number of African medical professionals through the 1940s. It also considers the multiple roles of biomedically trained African professionals in colonial and postcolonial West Africa.

Chapter 2 builds on this by highlighting the contributions of pharmacists in colonial and postcolonial Senegal. Relying on colonial records, university records, and newspaper articles, I show how the pharmacy field changed from predominately French and male to almost entirely African and significantly female. I consider the ways the pharmacy profession was embraced by West Africans, particularly by women, as they became established stakeholders in biomedical care by the late colonial period.

Chapter 3 highlights women as professionals and expands our understanding of women's access to property and formal lending structures, focusing on the second half of the twentieth century. I contribute to the literature on African women and development by arguing that not all African women are undereducated and have access only to local, informal credit schemes such as *tontines*.[14] In fact, I argue that female pharmacists have successfully entered into and risen in the formal financial sector to pursue professional opportunities, and I discuss their negotiations of entrepreneurship. Here I rely heavily on government legislation, the regulations of pharmaceutical associations, and the norms of the pharmaceutical profession, as well as discussions in interviews about pharmacists' access to credit. In addition, I assess how the devaluation of the CFA franc and the importation of large amounts of pharmaceuticals have affected pharmacy entrepreneurship. Finally, I examine some family relationships among pharmacists and how they helped some women open pharmacies.

Chapter 4 examines the importance of familial, social, and professional cultural norms in succeeding as a pharmacist in postcolonial Senegal. I begin by broadly contextualizing the major obstacles to professional success and examining organizational policies and politics, the effects of pharmacy proliferation, and the impact of the fact that most pharmaceuticals are imported. Analyzing both official documents and interviews, I present thorough profiles of selected pharmacists, including their background, status, and ethnicity. Drawing from oral narratives, official papers, and ideas about marriage and divorce in Senegal, I also explore how women's educational and economic success impacts nuclear and extended family relations.

Chapter 5 highlights the implications of the long-established illegal pharmaceutical trade and details its expansion in the latter decades of the twentieth century. It has always been a major challenge for government officials and medical practitioners. Beginning with developments in the 1940s and 1950s and relying on public records, oral testimony, and personal observation, I chronicle the growth of this market in French West Africa as well as transformations in postcolonial Senegal, to highlight its connection to a larger global trade. I also assess some of the key players, institutions, and cities involved in it. This chapter is critical to a larger understanding of the intersection of globalization and public health policy in colonial and postcolonial contexts. It shows how pharmacists responded to these challenges through individual initiative and collective action as well as through interactions with clients and the government.

The concluding chapter reaffirms the significant role played by biomedically trained pharmacists in Senegal. It emphasizes the need to understand the connections between professional growth, gender, and entrepreneurship in Senegal's pharmacy sector. Considering the dearth of material on African medical professionals, and on pharmacists in particular, the importance of this book, the first historical study of Senegal's pharmacists, is unmatched. Further, as the first project to recognize and focus on the increasing role of women pharmacists, this study offers indispensible insight into African women's access to property and their changing role in society.

1 France's Biomedical Expansion: Creating African Medical Personnel

Science knows no country, because knowledge belongs to humanity, and is the torch which illuminates the world.

—Louis Pasteur

Throughout the twentieth century, Senegal was at the intersection of indigenous, Islamic, and Western medical knowledge. This predominately Muslim, Francophone West African country embodied the notion of science without borders. Furthermore, the establishment of the School of Medicine and Pharmacy in French West Africa early in the century transformed the practice of medicine and ideas about health and healing. This school led to the creation of a new professional class of African medical personnel. This professional class continued to expand during the course of the twentieth century and became an integral part of health care in postcolonial Senegal. In this chapter, I examine the intersections of French colonial expansion and African medical professionalization in French West Africa in the early to mid-twentieth century.

Precolonial Health Systems

In precolonial times, many African societies had complementary healing traditions that utilized herbal medicine in conjunction with different forms of religious intercession. Indigenous healing traditions were often complex practices involving plants, other materials, and rituals. These healing techniques were transmitted from generation to generation through oral traditions and apprenticeship. During this precolonial era, many Africans valued their health and well-being and judged political leaders and healers by their ability to protect their constituents and their community. Indigenous healers or intercessors invoked supernatural aid to ensure bountiful harvests, secure boundaries, and robust communities.[1]

Throughout the globe, humans have always tried to heal illness, pain, injury, and imbalance. The African continent was no exception, and healers were found in communities throughout Africa. Some of the most prominent caregiving figures in traditional medicine were the *sangomas* in South Africa, Zar intermediaries in Northeast Africa, and a variety of mediums along the Bight of Benin in West Africa. Numerous scholars have documented indigenous West African healing practices, most notably among the Igbo, Yoruba, Wolof, and Tuareg ethnic communities.[2] In many of these sub-Saharan societies, healing was holistically conceptualized as creating harmony between a person's physical and spiritual selves. In addition, healing often meant restoring balance with an ill person's family, community, and perhaps ancestors.[3] Most African healers employed both herbal and ritual methods of healing. Maghan Kéita suggests that "the gris-gris, the talisman, the amulet, had been a source of religious and medical power throughout Africa long before the inception of Islam."[4] Local ideas about healing were transcultural and included multifaceted approaches to the preservation and improvement of health. Indeed, traditional healing included herbs, spirit possession, gris-gris (talismans), and religious intercessions of different origin.

The spread of Islam in the West African subregion brought new ideas about healing and disease. Islam spread in Senegal from the ninth century. Many of its early adherents were clerics, merchants, and members of the ruling class. Large numbers of the masses converted in the eighteenth and nineteenth centuries, and Islamic ideas about religion and healing were often syncretized with existing health care traditions. Responses to disease varied according to whether the disease's origin was considered natural or supernatural.

Because African approaches to healing were already polycultural, Muslim therapeutic methods were usually complementary and did not rival biomedical treatments. In addition, both indigenous and Islamic ideas about healing were more holistic and less focused on the treatment of symptoms than were European medical "cures." Treatments for illness varied widely, and included Qur'anic recitations and religious intercessions (such as those performed by Wolof marabouts in Senegal), intercessions that relied on plant and animal products, herbal medicine, and spirit possession. In Senegal, the Serer, Wolof, Lébou, and Fula ethnic groups all employed local healing traditions.

In Western Europe, hospitals and universities began to flourish in the twelfth and thirteenth centuries.[5] Formal medical training was instituted at universities in Paris and Montpellier beginning in 1220.[6] As in Africa, medical knowledge in Europe was influenced by that of other regions. As Europeans gained greater knowledge of the globe through exchange, exploration, and conquest, they developed a broad body of medical knowledge. Plant-based *materia medica* was imported from the Americas, Southeast Asia, and Africa. As many of the biomedically trained pharmacists interviewed for this project pointed out, a high percentage of biomedical drugs were derived from plants. Apothecaries in the thirteenth century worked in tandem with doctors to provide drugs to patients. Senegal, influenced by both Islamic healing traditions and European biomedicine, was at the intersection of healing modalities. Both traditions would remain important through the colonial era.

The introduction of European biomedical practices to colonial Africa fundamentally changed indigenous approaches to healing. In Europe, medical personnel were increasingly trained in hospitals and universities, and these institutions incorporated medical experimentation, extensive research, and publication. European biomedical knowledge expanded exponentially in the seventeenth, eighteenth, and nineteenth centuries with new developments in germ theory, pharmaceuticals, and responses to epidemics. European physicians and other medical personnel believed their interventions were far superior to indigenous and Muslim practices, partly because they were more logical. Although practitioners of the biomedical approach competed with African health care practitioners, complementary health systems continued to exist in tandem with these imported healing traditions. Steven Feierman explores the diverse factors that contribute to diagnosis, healing, and medicine in Africa and argues that "in most African communities several types of healers work side by side: physicians or medical assistants, specialists in sorcery or spirit possession, Christian or Muslim religious healers, and others."[7] In Senegal, over time, patients became impressed with the results of biomedical approaches. Many of them conferred with both biomedical and religious healers, sometimes simultaneously for the same illness. In the colonial era, health care providers and pharmacists were aware of this practice and considered these factors in their interactions with clients. As a result, these two healing approaches are not mutually exclusive and often influence each other.

Indeed, the multiple Senegalese medical systems, some of indigenous origin and others imported from the West, are often more complementary than competing. For example, when I asked informants about indigenous and biomedical pharmacopeias, most discussed the influence of plant-based remedies on biomedical pills, tinctures, and the like. One pharmacist, Aïssatou Moreau, spoke to the historical connections of traditional healing: "Yes, I think that we should further develop pharmacopeia because our grandparents did not take medicine [biomedical drugs]. They healed themselves well for years with roots and plants. In my opinion, I would like more collaboration between pharmacists and people who practice pharmacopeia. However, this is rare here. At the university, there is a branch that considers these linkages."[8] Some pharmacists sold herbal medicines, and others agreed with Madame Moreau that biomedical and traditional health care practitioners should collaborate. The majority of my respondents supported a policy of marketing proven herbal remedies and creating a network of reputable traditional health practitioners. Like most of the world, Senegal has no system for certifying and regulating either herbal drugs or traditional healers.

Questions about the intentions of French and, later, black African doctors grew in parallel with French colonial health policy. France's attempts to curb epidemics and promote urban development, often by further subjugating African populations, were skeptically received. French authorities devalued African-owned property, black bodies, and African traditions, and disregarded traditional non-European ideas about health and sanitation in favor of their own theories of contagion. Some of the colonial health policies helped reduce the transmission of disease, but others promoted racial segregation and fostered illness.

Expansion of French Colonial Medicine

During the seventeenth century, France continued building medical facilities, but it also began laying the foundation for policy concerning the health of nonwhites. As early as 1685, France created a public health force to help prevent disease transmission within and between black and white communities in Martinique. From the eighteenth to the early twentieth centuries, the French colonial authorities promoted biomedical techniques and constructed medical establishments as part of France's global imperial colonizing mission. These medical establishments were established primarily to provide health care for European patients; auxiliary clinics and "native" hospitals were built to meet the needs of indigenous populations. The growth of France's overseas biomedical colonial mission connected its disparate colonies. Many of the architects of this mission spent time as colonial bureaucrats, leading to the cross-fertilization of policy connecting the Americas, Africa, Asia, and the Pacific.

France's biomedical policy in Africa was an integral part of its larger colonial policy. As many scholars have illustrated, France attempted to control disease through urban planning, segregation, quarantine, and preventive medicine.[9] Saint-Domingue received special treatment in an imperial ordinance of 1763 that required a series of investments in the colony, mandating the establishment of "a chief of colonies, three doctors, [and] a pharmacist," as well as other health care initiatives.[10] During the next few decades (including after the Haitian revolution), France continued to promote improvements in Saint Domingue's public health system. In Senegal, sustained expansion of biomedicine began in the eighteenth and nineteenth centuries. As early as 1770, authorities planned to establish a surgeon at Saint-Louis and Gorée to provide medical assistance to French workers. In 1787, in response to growing epidemics, plans were developed to create a new hospital to care for the infirm.[11] The hospital was constructed in Saint-Louis between 1820 and 1829.

Between 1850 and 1900, Senegal had two military hospitals, a colonial hospital, a service to import and distribute pharmaceuticals, and a growing contingent of French medical personnel.[12] The first pharmacy was established in Senegal in 1882.[13] This date is significant. The pharmacy profession was expanding in the Western world, and many cities were starting to cultivate pharmacists. During this period, France also began informally training African workers to assist in medical affairs. In addition, Africans who came from the four communes of Saint-Louis, Gorée Island, Dakar, and Rufisque were allowed access to French public health services.

Colonial Medical Personnel

From 1890 to the end of the colonial period, a small contingent of colonial pharmacists managed pharmacy in France's overseas territories. The remaining colonial pharmacists worked in tropical medicine laboratories in France. They helped to develop breakthroughs in germ theory, vaccination, and biomedical drug preparation, which in turn helped promote public health both overseas and at home. Their training included courses in chemistry, biology, and toxicology at the School of Health Services for Colonial Troops (Pharo) in Marseille and at the School of Medicine and Pharmacy in Bordeaux. Pharmacists finished their training with an internship at the Michel-Lévy hospital in Marseille.[14] Physicians were trained in Bordeaux at the School of Naval Health as well as at Pharo. Once trained, they were prepared to provide a variety of services in their colonial posts.

Colonial pharmacists, like their postcolonial counterparts, engaged in a variety of professional functions. They worked as administrators in colonial hospitals, in pharmacies, and in laboratories. Many also taught African auxiliaries and other students at the medical school. A select few served as pharmacy inspectors, a coveted role in the colonial medical service. In addition, their biomedical training in chemistry and other sciences was especially important. The French government firmly regulated who could practice pharmacy in the colony; in French West Africa, a pharmacist had to have a French diploma and pass an examination. Where there were no pharmacies, doctors were authorized to sell medicine.[15]

Pharmacists provided diagnoses, prepared syrups and serums, measured dosages, supervised African personnel, and managed inventory. This latter duty was very important, because they were often stationed in hot, humid climates with unreliable electricity and limited equipment. Supplies were often ordered months in advance, but because of the distance between the metropole and the colony, they sometimes never arrived or arrived in unusable condition. Medical personnel occasionally had to make do with what they had. For example, a prominent colonial medical doctor, Albert Calmette, substituted Asian water buffalo for pigs in tests for the Pasteur Institute.[16] Substitutions were used in preparing insulin serums, and penicillin was recuperated from urine to be used again. In addition, shea, mango, and other local seed butters were used in place of pomades.[17]

Jean-François Le Blanc worked as a doctor and professor of surgery in France and Cameroon. He served in rural Cameroon in the 1950s, where he ran the only clinic in a five-hundred-kilometer radius. Because of the huge demand for medical care and the limited staff and supplies, he functioned as both specialist and generalist.[18] Like his colonial compatriots in other parts of the global South, he resorted to creativity and innovation to manage his clinic. When supplies ran low, for instance, he had his secretary buy thread in the market to use in surgeries. Innovation at both public and private levels was critical to the growth of medical practice and research in France's empire.

Several prominent pharmacists emerged from France's overseas colonial ranks, and most of them spent time working in French West Africa. Beginning in 1936, Eugène Le Floch worked in Guinea, Chad, and Cameroon, as well as at posts in Indochina. Félix Busson completed his degree at Pharo after working in the military during World

War II. Busson was a major figure in colonial French West Africa and spent considerable time in Senegal, where he served as head pharmacist for Dakar's Dantec Hospital from 1950 to 1953.[19] He continued his career with several posts in Asia and Africa. Another prominent pharmacist was Gauthier Pille, who worked in Madagascar and Chad before moving to Dakar. In the 1950s and 1960s, Pille held a variety of positions in Dakar, working as head pharmacist at Dantec Hospital, holding a university professorship, and codirecting a food science laboratory.

Entry and Growth of African Health Care Officials

France's colonial expansion between 1870 and 1918 brought many challenges; one was how to manage overseas medical expansion. In response, France consolidated its overseas medical facilities and personnel. In 1890, an overseas branch of the Pasteur Institute opened in Saigon, followed by others in Madagascar (1901), Congo (1910), and Senegal (1913).[20] Several microbiology and chemistry labs, scientific missions, hospitals, and other facilities were established during this period as well. Pharmacies also spread in the French colonies during the nineteenth century, and one was established in Senegal by the 1880s.[21] This consolidation and expansion of medical facilities was part of a larger development effort (*mise en valeur*), and significant investment was made in medical facilities and training in French West Africa. Despite habitual siphoning of funds for other projects, major cities in French West Africa became some of the leading providers of health care in sub-Saharan Africa. If they had been allowed to flourish to their full potential, their legacy might be better known today.

In the late nineteenth and early twentieth centuries, France faced a series of disease epidemics in its colonies. Senegal endured a major outbreak of yellow fever in Saint-Louis in 1878 and suffered bubonic plague outbreaks beginning in 1914. Smallpox, influenza, and meningitis were also common during this period. These recurring epidemics were critical to France's approach to medical planning in French West Africa. In July 1914, at a conference of the Local Hygiene

Committee, William Ponty, governor general of French West Africa, and other French administrators agreed to demolish buildings and enforce residential segregation in an attempt to reduce transmission of the bubonic plague.[22] These efforts led to the creation of Medina, a segregated African ghetto near the center of Dakar. By August, approximately three thousand people were living there.

At the same time, elections were being held for the French Chamber of Deputies. Blaise Diagne, the Senegalese candidate, was the first African elected to the French assembly. In the next few years, Diagne became an important intermediary between France and Africa on medical policy.

Nascent medical infrastructure coupled with developments in politics and health care helped to ensure the final stages of France's "medical penetration" of French West Africa. French military medical personnel in the colonies were strained, because of their limited numbers. In 1912, forty-two medical doctors were stationed in French West Africa, an increase of only nine since the last decade of the nineteenth century.[23] In 1905, Ernest Roume, then governor general of French West Africa, established the Indigenous Medical Assistance (Assistance médicale indigène, AMI), and this was followed by the appointment of African medical assistants and the founding of a hospital for African patients in 1913.[24]

The desire to establish a school of medicine in French West Africa stemmed from the 1912 annual report of the inspector of civil health services for the French colonial missions.[25] Interest in training African medical personnel had increased in the late nineteenth century, and the creation of the AMI facilitated training West Africans to implement France's biomedical policy. However, the 1914 bubonic plague outbreak and World War I postponed the opening of the school. Moreover, the Spanish influenza pandemic immediately after the war killed more people globally than the war itself. Colonial administrators were spurred to begin more advanced training of African personnel.

Disease epidemics, low numbers of French personnel, and economic losses from the war all culminated in a greater desire on the part of colonial administrators for a school of medicine. In an article published in 1920 Dr. Aristide Le Dantec, the school's first director, described how the war caused the French government to better "appreciate [its] colonial domain" and to utilize the "labor of the natives."[26] Le Blanc also described the impact of World War I on France's colonial medical policy. He contended that the economic blow of the war meant that existing medical facilities and manpower were insufficient to meet the demand. For example, the hospital that he managed in Cameroon had only thirty medical beds, with another fifteen designated for maternity.[27] To fill this need, indigenous medical clinics and mobile health care expanded, and local auxiliary workers were trained. Ultimately the goal was to reduce the number of French colonial doctors in the field. This policy had been successful in the colonial settings of Vietnam and Madagascar and was now being implemented in French West Africa.

The Jules Carde African School of Medicine (later the School of Medicine and Pharmacy, and now part of Cheikh Anta Diop University) was finally established in Dakar in 1918. During the following year, a section for training pharmacists was added, with sections subsequently created in Dakar, Senegal, and Bamako, Mali (School of Veterinary Science), to train nurses, midwives, and veterinarians. By 1930, French West Africa had facilities to train all types of medical professionals. Senegal was one of the first places where Africans had access to European biomedical training. The British opened facilities to train African medical personnel in 1923 (Uganda), 1924 (Sudan), and 1930 (Nigeria).[28] In Senegal, the initial terms of study were four years for doctors, three years for pharmacists and midwives, and two years for nurses. During the early decades of medical professionalization, Senegalese medical personnel were considered auxiliary unless they completed further study abroad. The creation of the African School of Medicine in 1918 helped ensure the success of biomedical expansion in French West Africa.

Educating African Medical Personnel

The 1870s and 1880s were an important period in the development of French colonial policy. Responding to France's defeat in the 1870–71 Franco-Prussian War, French officials, media, and academics promoted colonial expansion, which led to the growth of colonial education initiatives. The diffusion of the French language was one of France's primary imperial goals. In Africa, colonial authorities believed that men would spread the language in public spaces while women used it in private spaces and taught it to their children. Authorities also hoped to create a group of Africans who, by mastering French linguistic and cultural mores, would become cultural intermediaries between France and the native inhabitants of the colonies. This was the reason for the creation of Senegal's four communes: Saint-Louis (1872), Gorée Island (1880), Rufisque (1880), and Dakar (1887). The communes were a unique feature of colonial Senegalese history. In creating an African intermediary class, France advocated personal assimilation and personal association. Mamadou Diouf argues that "assimilation did not reduce areas of innovation and creativity available to the colonized."[29] Similar notions of hybridization were found throughout the African Diaspora. Globally, people of African descent who were either politically colonized or marginalized often created new sociocultural norms and rituals in response to new realities.

By the opening of the twentieth century, France had consolidated its power into distinct regions. In North Africa, it controlled areas that are now Algeria, Morocco, and Tunisia. French West Africa, with its power base in Senegal, stretched from modern Mauritania to Burkina Faso. In the center of the continent, the French consolidated their power under the name of French Equatorial Africa. In addition to these colonies and several island territories, France also absorbed a few German colonies in Africa after the war.[30]

The colonial archives describe the mission of educating not only male medical professionals but also their female counterparts. The creation of the medical school in 1918 and of the pharmacy and midwifery programs in 1919, coupled with the opening of the Rufisque Girls' School (École normale des jeunes filles de Rufisque) in 1938, led to the growth of education for women and girls. Education was a critical part of the French civilizing mission, and the combination of education and public health policy helped to serve two purposes. In 1920, Aristide Le Dantec spoke of the goal of giving "youth of both sexes" access to education in order to promote a "harmonious equilibrium of intellectualism and morality in future [African] families."[31] The Rufisque Girls' School prepared women and girls (ages thirteen to twenty) for careers in midwifery and teaching; it laid the foundation for a professional class of Senegalese women. In its first year it enrolled forty-six students, of whom thirty-three were Christian and eleven Muslim. Daniel Ouezzin Coulibaly described the challenges of recruiting female students: "If the indigenous population hesitates to send their girls to our schools it is because they are afraid that they will receive an emancipated child who does not respect authority and who after many years of study appears lazy and likes a life of luxury."[32] Coulibaly was able to draw on his experiences as a West African man and colonial bureaucrat to gain a nuanced glimpse into the challenges faced by female African students. If a woman was educated and exposed to values that conflicted with those of her family and community, it was often difficult for her to return to the community. Coulibaly proposed that the government carefully consider these issues and ensure that the Rufisque Girls' School fully supported its graduates.

In addition, because female students arrived at the school with less preparatory education than did males, the midwifery curriculum was much less stringent than those of other medical fields. Students were taught basic hygiene, infant care, basic anatomy of a pregnant woman, and obstetrics.[33] The rationale for training African midwives was to lower infant and maternal mortality rates and to transfer some of the burden of infant care from colonial officials to more specialized medical professionals. In the 1920s and 1930s, four French midwives were stationed in Dakar and one was stationed in Abidjan.[34]

The opening of the School of Medicine in November 1918 coincided with the expansion of local medical facilities, including maternity wards, pharmaceutical dispensaries, and sanatoria. Medical students were initially chosen by a committee from the William Ponty School, one of the premier secondary institutions of learning in French West Africa. In return for their training, the students had to commit to "serving ten years in the cadre of indigenous medical assistant services in the French West Africa" regional administrative branch.[35] According to a legislative decree by Charles de Gaulle in 1944, students could explore other options after spending ten years in colonial service. African personnel who wanted to practice privately had to request authorization from the commissioner of the colonies.[36]

A section for training pharmacists was added to the medical school in 1919. In the beginning, French bureaucrats had difficulty recruiting African pharmacy students. Students were more interested in studying medicine than pharmacy.[37] Many of the early pharmacists were not able to open pharmacies, for a variety of reasons. Regulations strictly limited the number of pharmacies and required a minimum distance between them. In addition, the requirement to spend ten years in colonial service prompted many African graduates to pursue other professional opportunities instead of waiting ten years to open their own pharmacies. After graduation, most African pharmacists worked as salaried personnel in privately owned pharmacies or in other medical contexts.

Upon opening the school, the minister of the colonies, Henri Simon, had set out the goals that the French colonial administration hoped to achieve in establishing Western medical training in Africa: "The service of the [indigène] of French West Africa is good for the operation . . . as well as the social and economic future of this group of colonies. . . . The indigenous doctors, trained in our practices . . . and hygienic methods . . . are destined to combat major epidemics that rage in this part of our colonial domain."[38] Further, the school's records mention the hope that African medical personnel would, through French training, develop a "professional conscience" modeled on French notions of health care.[39]

The French authorities tightly controlled the School of Medicine and Pharmacy. Admission was capped each year, and students were required to be between eighteen and twenty-five, to pass an entrance exam, and to submit letters of recommendation from medical personnel, as well as providing identification and proof of sound academic standing.[40] Medical training for African personnel was fairly rigorous. Students were required to take numerous classes in the physical sciences. In addition, they held internships at local hospitals and other medical facilities. Several tracks of biomedical training were available. For example, to earn nomination to the position of "principal doctor, pharmacist, or midwife," students were required to intern for three months at the principal hospital and pass a two-tier examination administered by high-level public health administrators.[41] Further, practice of the pharmacy profession was strongly regulated. The director of the Public Health Service, Colonel Garcin, explained to the director general of the interior that, according to a 1926 decree, "no one can practice the pharmacy profession, open a pharmacy, prepare, sell, or exchange any goods for medicine in French West Africa if he is less than 25 years old, has not completed a degree in pharmacy granted by the French government, and passed exams administered by colonial government."[42]

During the colonial period, enrollment at the School of Medicine and Pharmacy varied by discipline. According to Louis Couvy, an administrator for the French colonial health services, 97 auxiliary doctors, 150 auxiliary midwives, and 15 auxiliary pharmacists had graduated by 1930.[43] Despite the support it had shown for the school prior to its creation, the state provided mixed support once it was established. It had been decreed that the school would receive substantial financial payments from the metropole. However, in practice it was funded from the budget of French West Africa, without any direct support from Paris.[44] Many instructors and students responded creatively to this lack of support at higher government levels and the resulting shortages of resources. The colonial instructors at the school had to employ the improvisational skills that many had used as practicing medical professionals in the colony.

The curriculum at the School of Medicine and Pharmacy was abbreviated during the early years, with initial terms of three and four years of study that were similar to those for a bachelor's degree or advanced technical training. Despite this brevity, the graduates of these programs were extensively trained in the field and in local hospitals and clinics. The rigor and length of the curriculum meant that few students completed their training; between 1922 and the early 1940s three or fewer students graduated from the pharmacy program per year, although several more were admitted.[45] In these decades, the French colonial government supported medical students with stipends, meals, and uniforms.[46] Students had to manage their own meals during holidays, but students who wanted to travel received funding from colonial budgets. Medical and pharmacy students had similar curriculums, with medical students undergoing instruction that was more specialized and longer. For example, pharmacy students took a variety of chemistry and biological science courses as well as courses geared toward pharmaceutical practice. Medical students took chemistry and biology courses, but also ones in hygiene, epidemiology, obstetrics, ophthalmology, advanced French, and physics, as well as several clinical courses. Students in both tracks were required to intern in clinical settings in the final years of instruction. In contrast, the midwifery program was less rigorous, reflecting the students' lower levels of educational preparation. Much of their curriculum centered on general instruction in linguistics, mathematics, and skills associated with females, such as sewing.[47]

In addition to the colonial archives, published and unpublished material by medical professionals also provides a glimpse into the historical development of medical education in French West Africa. Two pharmacists, Rito Alcantara and Majhemout Diop, wrote about their experiences as students in the 1940s, and Birago Diop, a veterinarian, and Aoua Kéita, a midwife, chronicled their experiences in the 1920s and 1930s and the 1950s, respectively. Alcantara spent three years in Montpellier, where he completed his studies in pharmacy in 1948. (During the colonial era and early postcolonial period, a degree in pharmacy obtained in the colony was equivalent to the same degree earned in France.) He enjoyed his studies and the time he spent socializing with students from other parts of the French colonial empire. He describes his time in Montpellier as "three beautiful years . . . that were enriching and unforgettable." The only academic difficulty he faced was in chemistry, which he had not studied for a number of years.[48]

After completing his studies, Alcantara returned to Senegal, where he worked as assistant pharmacist to Henri Guigon. Guigon, a French national, had opened his pharmacy, originally called Moderne, in Dakar in 1935.[49] Because Alcantara had studied in France and not in Senegal, he was exempt from the requirement of colonial service. As a result, within a year he had established his own pharmacy, Pharmacie Africaine, which opened on 19 October 1949.[50]

In *Mémoires de luttes,* Majhemout Diop described his experience as a student at the African School of Medicine and Pharmacy during the 1940s. He initially wanted to study not pharmacy but medicine, but his paternal aunt decided that he should study pharmacy, and he complied. He described the training as strict, like military discipline. The challenging curriculum led some students to withdraw and others to take a long time to complete their training. In 1947, their third and final year, Diop's class had eleven students, but he was the only one to receive a diploma. During his third-year internship at the Dantec Hospital, he worked under the supervision of Pierre Fayemi, a well-respected pharmacist whose children later practiced medicine and pharmacy. Diop admired Fayemi and other older pharmacists, such as Dr. Francis d'Almeida and Dr. Matheiu, who were established medical professionals in Dakar.[51]

After completing his medical studies, Diop completed studies in other disciplines. In 1973, almost thirty years after graduating from the School of Medicine and Pharmacy, he completed a doctorate at the Institute of African Studies in Moscow. His two-volume *Histoire des classes sociales dans l'Afrique de l'Ouest* (History of Social Classes in West Africa) was based on his thesis.[52] After completing his doctorate, he returned to Africa and worked as a social science researcher in Bamako, Mali. Because of his initial reluctance to become a pharmacist and his long-term political conflict with the Senegalese state, Diop did not practice for decades. He opened his pharmacy in Dakar in 1977, thirty years after receiving his degree. Alcantara's and Diop's stories are particularly important because these men grappled with the difficulties of professional practice in the transition from the late colonial period into the postcolonial era.

Aoua Kéita, a native of Mali, was one of the first women to study at the Girls' Preparatory School in Bamako, Mali. She found this opportunity an honor and says that it "was by the grace of God that the French created a girls' school in Bamako." Like many of the women of her generation, she faced social pressure not to attend school, and her mother found it "scandalous" that her daughter was enrolled. After completing her early education, Kéita moved to Dakar, where she studied midwifery from 1928 to 1931. Her training was rigorous, and she interned at the Dantec Hospital, where she made the rounds every morning. After completing her training in midwifery, Kéita was immediately transferred back to Mali, where she would begin work as a midwife for the colonial government in Gao.[53] Kéita's reminiscences are critical in reconstructing the voices of women medical professionals in the colonial period.

After graduating high school, Birago Diop decided that he wanted to study medicine. In 1928 he began studying nursing in Saint-Louis through the assistance of Frédéric Houillon, the director general of French West Africa. However, he decided that he wanted to continue his studies in France, and with the help of Blaise Diagne, he was able to obtain a scholarship to study at the National Veterinary School of France in Toulouse. This was the only scholarship available from the office of the governor general of French West Africa at this time. He found his courses in biology less challenging than zoology. In addition, one of his zoology professors, Mr. Wendel, offered engaging lectures; Diop describes them as "quasi-poetic and rhythmic." In November 1933, he received his doctorate in veterinary studies and went to practice veterinary medicine in Maisons-Alfort, near Paris. Birago Diop's experiences in France were similar to those of Rito Alcantara. During his four years in France, Diop spent time with many students from Senegal, French West Africa, the Antilles, and France. Many of these alliances and friendships continued throughout his lifetime, bolstering professional and political connections. Diop also met his wife, Marie-Louise Paule Pradère, in France; they were married in Toulouse in 1934.[54]

Finally, Félix Houphouët-Boigny (future president of Côte d'Ivoire) studied medicine in Dakar. After completing his studies at William Ponty, he expressed his interest in becoming a doctor. The

African School of Medicine had recently opened and, with the support of one his instructors, Claude Raquin, Houphouët-Boigny enrolled in 1921.[55] While there, he formed friendships and associations with African students from different parts of French colonial Africa, and he also made connections with some prominent colonial officials, including Aristide Le Dantec.

What is particularly interesting is that while these medical professionals came from different national and class backgrounds, they all were influenced by the political changes brewing at the time. Majhemout Diop and Aoua Kéita became active politically as anticolonial activists and opposition leaders.[56] Birago Diop would later become an ambassador to several countries as well as a poet. Félix Houphouët-Boigny became the first president of Côte d'Ivoire, a position he held from 1960 to 1993. Finally, while Rito Alcantara never held political office, he became politicized during his time in France and was later quite active in professional politics.

As previously noted, strict numerical regulations kept many students from opening a pharmacy. The number of pharmacies allowed in all of Senegal was capped at thirty-three, but by 1945 several pharmacists were graduating from the African School of Medicine and Pharmacy each year. The significant number of pharmacies meant that native and expatriate European populations had access to pharmaceutical care.

The second phase in the evolution of the African School of Medicine and Pharmacy began in 1950, when it became a major component of the newly created Institute of Higher Education of Dakar. Faculty from the Universities of Paris and Bordeaux collaborated to steer this new institution. Some of them became full-time faculty members or administrators in Senegal, while others held temporary, part-year appointments. A number of French government officials attended the school's opening ceremonies on 13 November 1950. Accompanied by the school's director, Monsieur Camerlynck, the high commissioner of French West Africa, Paul Bechard, governor general of French West Africa, gave a few remarks. He began by saying, "Liberate yourselves from the inferiority complex born in the comparisons between French West Africa and the metropole. This school is the beginning of a future for its faculty and for their students. This school will offer the same level of instruction found in France with equivalent diplomas."[57]

Twelve years earlier, a lower-ranking bureaucrat had offered a contradictory perspective: "One is not able to escape the fact that [we] cannot give the same level of medical education to students in French West Africa . . . nor our classical culture, nor our intellectual evolution, as to European students."[58] Bechard's comments showed an evolution in French ideas about the education of Africans. Policymakers had moved from earlier ideas of African medical personnel as auxiliaries to seeing them as fully credentialed medical professionals who were trained in the same manner as their French counterparts. Bechard's comments—in spite of their patriarchal tone—were earnest and led to the relocation of the School of Medicine to a facility adjunct to the African hospital in Dakar and adjacent to the university. Other reforms included an expansion of requirements for the degree.

The Institute of Higher Education became the University of Dakar in 1957. In 1962, the School of Medicine became the university's faculty of medicine and pharmacy, with departments for medicine, pharmacy, and dentistry. With these changes came additional requirements for entry into medical study. Students were now required to have a college background before entering the faculty of medicine and pharmacy. In addition, the length of the medical degree programs had increased. Pharmacy students were now required to study for five years and spend the sixth writing a dissertation. The first doctoral degrees were awarded in 1962. Medical professionals from French West Africa and postcolonial Francophone countries thus became more competitive in the global arena.

Colonial and Missionary Education in French West Africa

Early education—like more advanced medical studies—was sometimes fraught with competing cultural ideas. During the early colonial period, Dakar's schools included a significant percentage of post-secondary students who were not Senegalese, or even African. After France's consolidation of political power and the early twentieth-century reforms in colonial West Africa, one-third of all Senegalese students attended schools in Dakar. Dakar's schools attracted students from throughout French West Africa and also taught children of French colonial officials. Until the 1940s and 1950s, the student population was ethnically, racially, and regionally diverse. During the first twenty years of independence, these demographics shifted, until the majority of students in Senegalese schools were Senegalese themselves.

Before the colonial era, West African education was influenced by both local and imported, mostly Islamic, modes of knowledge production. Even as Western forms of knowledge were reproduced in the colony, Islamic education, in the form of Qur'anic schools, continued to persist. In the nineteenth and twentieth centuries, most Senegalese children received some type of Qur'anic instruction in the pre-primary and early primary school years. Most of those who went on to receive a Western education continued their Qur'anic studies simultaneously with their early years of Christian or secular Western schooling.[59]

Missionaries pioneered the establishment of schools throughout sub-Saharan Africa. They opened the first boys' schools in Senegal in 1817 and the first girls' schools in 1822; secondary education was introduced in the 1840s. The first schools were established on Gorée Island and in Saint-Louis. Two of the largest proponents of missionary education were the Sisters of St. Joseph de Cluny and the Brothers of Ploërmel. Anne-Marie Javouhey, the French nun who founded the Sisters of St. Joseph de Cluny, was especially influential in the establishment and spread of girls' schools in Senegal. In her letters, she spoke of her desire to provide open schools for children while spreading Christian ideals.[60] Despite their efforts, however, missionaries were often not supported by the government, and the majority of their schools' funds came from church budgets.

The early decades of French educational policy included many false starts and resulted in high rates of teacher turnover. Colonial educational pedagogy focused on preparing students to speak well, as well as on reading, writing, and arithmetic. French ideas about hygiene were also promoted, especially at girls' schools, where home economics courses became a major part of the curriculum.

While missionary educational institutions gradually spread, they were met with ambivalence by the largely Muslim population. Student enrollment in the early decades was limited. One writer spoke of hopes for a new secular school in 1863: "The government has recently opened a secular school in Dakar in the hopes of attracting Muslim children, because it is said that their parents refused to send them to missionary schools, because they believe that the instructors will speak about religious conversion. At this school, they will not hear any of that, plus they will have other advantages . . . such as the European headmaster to teach French, and a marabout to teach them to read the Qur'an."[61] However, because the new secular school was close to a missionary-run school, locals considered it an extension of missionary education.

"The Colonizer and the Colonized"

While the transfer of biomedical knowledge to African medical professionals was relatively swift, it was not without complications. In French West Africa, this emerging professional class faced questions from religious authorities and from many of the inhabitants of the colonies. Like the Europeans who colonized them, Africans had to adjust to the expansion of biomedicine. Health care began to be broadly medicalized in France in the eighteenth century, but at the end of the nineteenth, the French still neither fully trusted nor accepted doctors. Traditional remedies existed alongside biomedical cures. Those living in rural areas were especially wary, and also faced the challenge of translating diagnoses and instructions from formal French into local languages.[62] As biomedical knowledge was expanding in the colonies, it was also expanding in the metropole, and biopolitics in the colony was inextricably tied to developments at home. Michel Foucault argues that state medicine was the first stage of the "formation of social medicine," and the final stage was "labor force medicine."[63] This was especially significant in the colony, as French medical personnel, together with the emerging African personnel, worked to prevent and eradicate disease, especially epidemic disease. One way of doing this was through residential segregation. In the major colonial cities, such as Dakar, Lagos, Nairobi, and Abidjan, most Africans were zoned to certain neighborhoods. Europeans often lived at higher elevations to avoid "pollution" or "contamination." At the same time, in Paris, the wealthy and the less privileged were moving into separate residential districts.[64] Much of the literature on urban planning and segregation in colonial Africa focuses primarily on African cities, failing to see the ways that urban planning in the colony was connected to the metropole. Scholars must seek out these the parallels to further interrogate nineteenth-century transnational urban health policy.

In *A Dying Colonialism* (*L'an cinq, de la révolution algérienne*), Frantz Fanon masterfully captures the tensions between the colonized, those who colonized, and those who practiced "colonial" medicine. Born in Martinique, Fanon studied medicine in France with a specialization in psychiatry. He practiced medicine while stationed in Algeria for several years, and his work in psychiatry featured prominently in his *Black Skin, White Masks* (*Peau noires, masques blancs*). He became politically radicalized after witnessing atrocities during the French-Algerian war, in which Algeria sought to break the colonial shackles and emerge as an independent state. *A Dying Colonialism* and the *Wretched of the Earth* (*Les damnés de la terre*) reveal his view of decolonization and native rule. Written in 1959, *A Dying Colonialism* firmly sided with the Algerians. Fanon was, in fact, so politicized that he joined the Algerian Nationalist Movement and advocated the liberation of colonized and marginalized peoples worldwide.

Despite this personal involvement in decolonization, he was able to remain objective in analyzing the early stages of decolonization in his writings. In *The Wretched of the Earth*, Fanon speaks to the colonial violence and national consciousness. He finds that "decolonization is always a violent phenomenon. . . . [It] is quite simply the replacing of a certain 'species' of men by another 'species' of men."[65]

Confronted with a world ruled by the settler, the native is always presumed guilty. But the native's guilt is never a guilt which he accepts; it is rather a kind of curse, a sort of sword of Damocles, for, in his innermost spirit, the native admits no accusation. He is overpowered but not tamed; he is treated as an inferior but he is not convinced of his inferiority. . . . He is in fact ready at a moment's notice to exchange the role of the quarry for that of the hunter. The native is an oppressed person whose permanent dream is to become the persecutor.[66]

Fanon's description of African desires after decolonization is also an accurate description of desires in the colony. Religious leaders, political figures, and many of the masses would question the motives of African medical professionals throughout the twentieth century.

As someone who grew up under French rule in Martinique, which had a different administrative status than did French possessions in either North or sub-Saharan Africa, Fanon himself faces an internal dilemma. Martinique was and is part of the *départements et territoires d'outre-mer,* France's overseas departments and territories. It has representatives in the French Parliament, and its inhabitants automatically receive French citizenship. It is evident in his writings that Fanon struggled with his race, class, and citizenship. *Black Skin, White Masks* makes clear that Fanon experienced racial prejudice while living in France. He deconstructed what it means to constantly live under the microscope of the "white gaze" and discussed the precarious position of the educated black and the "dualness" of blackness in social interactions.[67] Even when blacks attained professional success, Fanon lamented, they always had to be better than their white counterparts and could not make mistakes, to avoid shame.[68] Later, when practicing medicine, he found himself at the other end of the status spectrum. As his biographer David Macey wrote, "Although Fanon was very sensitive about being addressed as *tu* by whites, he did find himself 'slipping' into that very way of addressing North Africans. His spontaneous use of *tu* stemmed not only from his medical superiority, but also from his internalization of the hierarchy that made Martinicans superior to Arabs: they were *indigènes,* but *he* was an honorary *toubab,*" a white person or foreigner.[69] This is one of the dilemmas that Fanon faced as he navigated "blackness" and "whiteness" in the metropole and in different colonies.

In *A Dying Colonialism,* Fanon committed an entire chapter, "Medicine and Colonialism," to unraveling the ways that local populations responded to the intersections of allopathic healing practices and biomedical expansion. Fanon stated that Africans perceived Western medicine as an extension of colonial oppression: "The colonized perceives the doctor, the engineer, the schoolteacher, the policeman, the rural constable, through the haze of an almost organic confusion." This "haze" makes Africans ambivalent in engaging with health care practitioners, both European and African, especially during the first decades of biomedical expansion. French biomedical care was considered an inextricable part of colonial oppression. Moreover, many Africans found biomedical treatment unreliable and ineffective. In early efforts to supplement Western medicine with traditional healing, these feelings contributed to a cross-cultural disconnection that hindered communication between colonial doctors and African patients. Doctors found it frustrating when patients missed appointments and did not adhere to pharmaceutical guidelines. In return, patients coming from more holistic healing traditions questioned the power of drugs that had to be taken for a long time.[70]

People responded this way to colonial European and African medical officials throughout French West Africa, and all African medical professionals—doctors, pharmacists, midwives—faced this predicament. In her autobiography, *Femme d'Afrique,* Aoua Kéita spoke of this dilemma. She began her assignment in Gao, Mali, by imposing not only French ideas about health care but also Western ideas about cleanliness. "I attempted to reduce the filth and especially to prevent its augmentation. Beds and cradles with bed bug infestations were immediately disinfected and mosquito nets washed." Of course, her attempts to disinfect the maternity ward were driven by scientific ideas of bacteria and other microscopic disease organisms.

These new ideas about childbirth that she imposed on local communities were often met with disdain, as many of the birthing mothers
and their families were offended by Kéita's mannerisms. She was spo-
ken of in the town as a *toubab* who prevented people from enacting
traditional rituals for childbirth and other events.[71] These descrip-
tions are important because they reflect the conflicts faced by Africans who were trained in European medical traditions. Especially in
the early decades, African medical personnel who were promoting
what they thought was better public health were often shunned by
their compatriots. In some cases, this tension would remain insur-
mountable throughout the twentieth century.

These conflicts over education and worldview occurred at all levels
of education. Disagreements were especially heated regarding wom-
en's training and professional practice, and their relationship to the
larger community. The writer Maríama Bâ faced a dilemma like that
described by Coulibaly. Her uncle and grandparents largely opposed
her enrollment in the Rufisque Girls' School. They felt that primary
school education was adequate. The director of the school, Madame
Maubert, intervened to convince her family that Maríama had an
important opportunity and that she wanted her to continue her education. Her family complied and she was allowed to enroll and completed her studies to become a teacher in 1947. She spoke of the pres-
tige and honor that she gained as a graduate of the Rufisque Girls'
School.[72] Bâ's reminiscences provide valuable insight into young
women's experiences of colonial education in French West Africa.

Despite these tensions and conflicts, African communities began
to accept biomedical expansion in the early decades of the twentieth
century. Malik Sy and Cheikh Sidia Baba were two Muslim religious
leaders who were critical allies of France's colonial medical mission
in Senegal. They both implored their followers to adhere to French
ideas of biomedicine and to accept residential segregation as a way of
protecting public health. Sy went so far as to urge Africans to accept
vaccinations and to visit AMI clinics for medical consultations.[73]

Despite the support of indigenous leaders and the material expansion of French biomedical institutions, France failed to sway public
opinion. In 1913, when discussions about the creation of a medical

school were increasing, Sy underwent a successful cataract operation in Saint-Louis. This operation likely prompted Sy to revise his previous opinion that "modern Western medicine and Islam were not compatible."[74] But as Kalala Ngalamulume first highlighted in his dissertation on public health in Senegal, and Myron Echenberg confirms in *Black Death, White Medicine,* French colonial officials failed to take advantage of this coup to rally support for biomedical care. Only a minor colonial bureaucrat in Tivaouane, Senegal, acknowledged the potential significance of Sy's cure. If the success of the operation were properly publicized, he argued, it could be "good propaganda in favor of our interests."[75] In failing to do so, the French lost an early and critical opportunity to amass public support for biomedicine. Ngalamulume shows that events discovered in the colonial archives can not only be used to reconstruct the historical narrative; they can also suggest other possible outcomes, hinging on a minor shift in human behavior. This particular case is quite fascinating, and given the broader colonial policy on biomedical expansion, it is particularly surprising that Sy's surgery was virtually unknown to colonial policymakers.

In conclusion, the expansion of pharmacy in Senegal coincided with the expansion of French colonialism. Colonial authorities made the decision to train indigenous people as part of their policy of socializing Africans in European mores of hygiene and healing, as well as in hopes of controlling disease in the colonies. In addition, both World War I and World War II created a need for more health care workers. As France spread its biomedical technology throughout Africa and Asia, the introduction of these techniques was not without its challenges. Traditional healing practices, including religious ones, were entrenched in many Senegalese communities. In West Africa, the record shows that all types of treatment modalities coexisted. It is clear that the introduction of biomedical technology left an indelible mark of "Frenchness" on Senegal. As Fanon suggests, education was a part of the colonizing project; African medical personnel were socialized in European ideas about healing. They were also expected to help transform local ideas about health and healing.

In many ways, the development of pharmacy in Senegal followed the development and maturation of the profession in France. Training Africans to be health care workers was not without cultural challenges. This was especially true for women, whose training was often controversial. Their training proved to be one of the most interesting developments in Senegal's history. Ultimately, the decision to educate Africans created a professional class whose members would become leaders in industry and politics in the former colonies.

2 Practicing Pharmacy

Working as a pharmacist is a very complex profession; one
manages the needs of patients while staying abreast of new
scientific developments and administering personnel, accounting,
and technology.

—Antonin Fayemi

Medical practitioners in French West Africa began to professionalize
in the late nineteenth century, and the growth of the profession was
a major development of the twentieth century. Doctors, nurses, midwives, pharmacists, and assistants would help transform local ideas
about health, disease, and healing. This chapter examines the historical trajectory of pharmacists in colonial and postcolonial Senegal
and their changing views of their roles in Senegal's public health sector. In the second part of the book, I will highlight the role of gender
and professionalism among the internal and external forces that influenced these pharmacists' lives.

Throughout this period, African medical professionals became especially adept as cultural translators of biomedical care. They integrated the profession and continued to proliferate through the twentieth century. African medical professionals, especially pharmacists,
were at the forefront of the cultural intersection of biomedicine and
local ideas about health and healing. Even though most of them did
not use traditional healing techniques, they were aware of their significance to local people. They were raised in pluralistic communi-

ties and were able to translate between European ideas about health and healing and those of West Africa. They were also linguistic mediators, code-switching between conversations with their European counterparts and with their African clients. Solange Decupper discussed this linguistic strength:

> The other pharmacists, it is true, were old French pharmacists. But with us, this is our country. We have a better understanding of the language. We speak the language. We know people, and there is an existing dialogue between us [and other Senegalese citizens]. It was up to us to [advance the profession]; I do not think that the others could do it. . . . We were closer to our clientele. . . . We speak in Wolof, we explain in Wolof and respond to questions. This helps to give better advice.[1]

As Decupper illustrates, African medical personnel provided diagnoses, asked questions, and gave instructions in local languages. They also offered nuanced cultural translations of new ideas about healing. Finally, of course, they resembled their patients. For these reasons, they were gradually embraced by local communities. Pharmacists were especially important as scientific and cultural interlocutors because they increasingly worked on the front lines of health care. In Senegal, especially, they became critical to the field.

As more European pharmacists were assigned to or trained in French Africa, colonial officials began to regulate the proliferation of pharmacies more closely. In 1926, pharmacists had to be at least twenty-five, and they were required to have earned a diploma of pharmacy in France and passed state-administered exams. Only pharmacists could sell medicines. In addition to restricting who could own a pharmacy, the French government limited the number of pharmacies allowed in each region and city. A 1955 law allowed twenty in Dakar, three in Saint-Louis and in Kaolack, two in Ziguinchor and in Thiès, and one in Diourbel and in Rufisque.[2]

This law also restricted Abidjan, in Côte d'Ivoire, to ten pharmacies and suspended the creation of new public clinics there. Here we can see that Dakar was receiving more resources and development efforts. This occurred for a number of reasons. As the second capital of French West Africa (having replaced Saint-Louis in that role in 1902), Dakar held a large percentage of French administrative buildings as well as French personnel. Doubtless, colonial officials wanted to develop their own surroundings. They may also have daily witnessed the need for expanded facilities. Further, the sustained restrictions on the creation of new pharmacies helped French pharmacists to maintain a monopoly on pharmacy ownership.

Despite the colonial justifications for restricting the spread of pharmacies, some pharmacists supported greater access to pharmacy ownership. On 11 August 1955, A. Touffait wrote a letter to the high commissioner of French West Africa arguing that "the general challenge to the installation of locally owned pharmacies is due to the increase in pharmacists from France in the urban centers, whose presence risks not leaving a place for pharmacists from French West Africa to open pharmacies."[3] But although he called attention to the challenges facing local pharmacists, Touffait did not press the issue and ended his letter with a conciliatory appeal to the high commissioner.

Most of the Africans with pharmacy degrees were stationed in French Africa while they completed the ten years of service they owed to the colonial government. Others who were now eligible to practice pharmacy independently worked as pharmacy assistants or temporary pharmacists during the owner's leaves of absence. Most pharmacies were owned by French men such as Henri Guigon, but the numbers of French women and African men owning pharmacies were slowly growing. African women began to graduate from the School of Pharmacy during the 1940s, but few had the opportunity to open a pharmacy.[4] As we will see in chapter 4, gender and racial discrimination were among the reasons for this. Others included early misconceptions about women's right to own property and the stringent regulations on the location and number of pharmacies. Women's familial obligations made them less able than men to commit to ten years of colonial service in other countries. Both men and women played critical roles in the development of the profession, and their stories are critical to the history of pharmacy in Senegal.

Two of the most notable men in the profession were Rito Alcantara and Majhemout Diop.

Rito Alcantara: Pharmacist and Leader

Rito Alcantara was born in Cape Verde in 1924, and his parents emigrated to Senegal when he was two years old. He received Senegalese nationality and described himself as African or as Cape Verdean-Senegalese. After completing his degree in Montpellier, he returned to Senegal and quickly became an integral part of the local pharmacy profession. As noted in chapter 1, he briefly interned with Bernard Guigon and then opened his own pharmacy. By completing his degree in France, he avoided the requirement to first work for the French government. Few African pharmacists who were trained during the colonial period managed this feat. I believe this requirement of a lengthy commitment, along with their limited access to financial capital and the strict limits on the number of pharmacies, prevented many Africans from owning pharmacies during the colonial period. Alcantara said that, including himself, only two Africans owned pharmacies in Dakar in 1949. He was the fifth African to own a pharmacy in Senegal. The economist Samir Amin found that there were only ten African-owned pharmacies in the region between Dakar and Thiès around 1960.[5] French and Lebanese-descended pharmacists owned the majority of the pharmacies in Senegal until the 1970s.

Rito Alcantara felt a strong affinity for all of Africa, which is reflected in the name of his pharmacy: Pharmacie Africaine, or "African pharmacy." He opened it on 19 October 1949 and operated it for more than fifty years, until his death.[6] It became a landmark in Dakar and was one of the highest-grossing pharmacies in the country. Alcantara was able to employ several formally trained pharmacy assistants, a store manager, and other employees. He described how he came to study pharmacy:

Thanks to my father, I was able to finish my secondary studies before advancing to the university. . . . In 1941, I wanted to study polytechnic studies and I was told no. I also considered Sciences Po, and I received a similar response. My father said that France was at war with Germany and that it was not possible. He said, "Je ne veux pas envoyer mon enfant avec les Nazis" [I do not want to send my child to the Nazis]. When the time came, I decided to study chemistry, but my father chose pharmacy instead. . . . At the time, you did not say no to your father. I replied, "'Bien, papa,' et voila. Je ne regrette pas, je suis très contente. Je suis fier avec la pharmacie!" ["Yes, papa" and it was settled. I do not regret the decision, as I am very happy. I am proud to have studied pharmacy!][7]

During his more than five decades as a pharmacist, Rito Alcantara faced a number of difficulties and enjoyed a number of successes. His major challenges included the density of pharmacies, the influx of new pharmacies, and the illegal trade in pharmaceuticals. In his recollections, he noted that early in his career there was one pharmacy for every five thousand people in the area, and this figure later decreased to one pharmacy for each thousand people. Alcantara was also concerned with the large numbers of students who were completing pharmacy degrees each year. Many were unemployed or underemployed and did not have the means to open private pharmacies. Finally, he considered the *marché illicite* (illegal trade in pharmaceuticals) to be a growing problem, and acknowledged that it was attractive to customers: "A drug may cost a thousand CFA francs at the pharmacy but five hundred CFA francs over there. The drug [purchased on the street] may not contain the active ingredient."[8] Many health care providers consider this parallel drug market a scourge to the community. I examine it in depth in chapter 5.

Alcantara was glad to see access to generic drugs improving in Senegal, because he believed this would benefit disenfranchised populations. At a 1994 Rotary Club International meeting in Dallas, Texas, he spoke with an American pharmacist who invited him to visit his pharmacy in Dallas. He found the visit fascinating and recalled, "He told me that in the United States, generic drugs represent a large percentage of pharmaceutical sales. He sells more generic drugs than anything else." At age seventy-five, and after five decades of practicing pharmacy, Alcantara said that his strongest desire was to work toward national public health. "I am proud to be a pharmacist. I work for the public health of my country!"[9]

Alcantara's story is important, as he was one of the first pharmacists of African origin to establish a pharmacy in Senegal. Africans who gained medical credentials during this time faced a number of hurdles on their way to pharmacy ownership, including restrictions on the density of pharmacies, limited access to funding, and discrimination in the profession. In addition, the majority of African pharmacists were, unlike Alcantara, obligated to work for France's colonial bureaucracy for ten years before entering private practice. After completing that service, most of the early pharmacists continued to work for French institutions or entered other professional arenas. Only a very small minority of African pharmacists were able to open pharmacies during the colonial period.

Majhemout Diop: Pharmacist and Political Activist

Majhemout Diop was born three years before Rito Alcantara, and he received his degree two years earlier, in 1947. The trajectory of Diop's training and practice of pharmacy differed greatly from Alcantara's. Diop studied and practiced pharmacy out of necessity and did not have a strong passion for the profession. When asked what he liked most about pharmacy practice, he replied, "Rien" [Nothing]. Diop was unapologetic about how his status and income as a pharmacy owner helped to propel him toward his true passion: politics.[10]

Diop was born on 30 September 1922 in Saint-Louis, Senegal. His father worked as a colonial official, and his mother was a homemaker. In 1935, Diop's father died; his mother followed two years later, leaving Diop, aged fifteen, and his four siblings orphaned. The death of his parents kindled his desire to excel in his studies. His paternal aunt decided that he should study pharmacy. He was disappointed, as he had wanted to become a physician, but in his memoirs he suggests that he enjoyed his studies and his interactions with senior pharmacists. He completed his degree in 1947 and remarked in interviews that during this period the French dominated the profession. At the time of his graduation, he estimated, only five pharmacies were owned by people of Senegalese heritage. This seems likely to be accurate, given Samir Amin's research.

Until the 1960s and 1970s, as we have seen, state policy regulating the proliferation of pharmacies was very strict and sternly enforced. Though he began working for the colonial government in exchange for his pharmacy training, Diop longed to postpone this obligation and further his education. He applied for a government subvention but was not awarded it, and he had a difficult time working briefly in Gabon. He longed to work where he wanted, under his own authority. After a short career in colonial service, he submitted his resignation on 30 November 1950, in a letter that made evident his personal autonomy and defiance. He cited the denial of two scholarships and lack of response to his requests for meetings as the reasons for his resignation. His resignation was formally approved in 1952, ending his career in the civil service.[11] This was a step on his path to battling the Senegalese state and international policy that he believed detrimental to people of the global South.

After being officially removed from colonial service, Diop spent the next three decades working in France, Russia, and Mali as well as spending short periods of time in Senegal. While studying in Senegal and France, he encountered a number of established and emerging political leaders, including Abdoulaye Wade, Félix Moumié, Félix Houphouët-Boigny, and Cheikh Anta Diop. He was strongly influenced by the political activities of Cheikh Anta Diop, the French communist party, and Marcus Garvey. His interest in politics grew, and in 1957, he became a founding member of the African Independence Party (Parti africain de l'indépendance, PAI).[12] The independent Senegalese government, led by Léopold Sédar Senghor, considered the party subversive, and as a result of his fervent opposition to state policy, Diop was briefly imprisoned; he went into exile in 1960. In 1976, members of Senghor's cabinet approached him about returning to Senegal. They agreed to provide him with a government loan to open a pharmacy and offered him an opportunity to restore political legitimacy to the PAI.

Some criticized Diop for accepting this arrangement, but the compromise served both him and Senghor. The events of the 1960s had weakened the PAI, and Diop, now fifty-five years old, needed the economic stability that running a pharmacy would provide. Moreover, Diop liked the idea of collaborating with the state to "Africanize" the pharmacy sector, as a way of promoting African development by Africans. He opened his Pharmacie de la Nation in 1977. After sixteen years in exile—and thirty years after he earned his pharmacy degree—Diop was now not only a politician and academic but also a pharmacy owner and employer. For the rest of his life Diop, like Alcantara, worked in his pharmacy.[13]

These glimpses into the professional practice of Majhemout Diop and Rito Alcantara illustrate the experience of pharmacists who studied and worked during the colonial era. They were among a handful of pharmacists trained during the colonial era who were still alive and practicing in the late twentieth century. Both men had long careers, but colonialism loomed large in their development as professionals and citizens in Senegal. Their reminiscences, coupled with their published and unpublished writings, make this clear, adding an African voice to colonial documentation.

A number of changes occurred in the first two decades after Senegal's independence in 1960. The pharmacy profession was not exempt from them. Senegalese, like other Francophone West African medical professionals, were no longer bound by French colonial statutes to provide service to the colonial government. Pharmacists could now open a pharmacy as soon as they completed their studies, so long as they obeyed zoning laws and were able to secure the necessary capital. These new opportunities were not without their challenges. Until the 1970s, French expatriates owned many of Senegal's private pharmacies, especially those in Dakar. However, as French nationals returned to the metropole or retired and zoning laws were relaxed, Senegalese pharmacists gradually began to carve a foothold as pharmacy owners in their native land.

Studying and Practicing Pharmacy in the Postcolonial Era

Marie Laure Konate

Marie Laure Konate, owner of Pharmacie Patte d'oie, was born in Dakar; she completed her degree in 1972 and established her pharmacy in 1974. She is the mother of four children, and one of the few divorced pharmacists among my interviewees. Although she is one of the longest-practicing pharmacists, she is not especially active in professional associations. Over the course of her career, she observed a number of changes in the profession, including variations in work ethics, the proliferation of pharmacies and their changing locations, and reductions in the price of drugs, which she says were much more expensive at the beginning of her career and are more affordable now. However, although consumers have better access to drugs than they used to, pharmacy owners face challenges. They pay for and receive pharmaceuticals at regularly scheduled intervals. Some drugs, especially neurological drugs and vaccines, require refrigeration. Pharmacists are required to keep them in stock, but because the poor national infrastructure leads to periodic electrical outages they often spoil, costing the pharmacist money. Despite the challenges, she enjoyed her work and offered strategies for success in it. To maintain success, she said, pharmacy owners must "manage their finances well, be consistently present at their business, be vigilant in managing employees, compensate vendors and employees on time, and maintain good customer service." She really enjoyed interacting with customers, finding satisfaction when they returned to tell her of the success of a treatment.[14]

Antonin Fayemi

Born in 1955 to a pharmacist and a midwife, Antonin Fayemi bridges the gap between pharmacy practice in late colonial and postcolonial Senegal. His father, Pierre Fayemi, had an illustrious career during the colonial era. He worked in Senegal in different capacities, working at the Pasteur Institute and helping to establish a pharmacy in Saint-Louis. He also spent two years working in Val-de-Grace, France. He is best known for his time at the Pasteur Institute and his role as head pharmacist of Dantec Hospital. Antonin Fayemi's earliest memories include accompanying his father to work, and by age ten he knew that he would follow in his father's professional footsteps. "The reason I became a pharmacist is very simple—because my father is a pharmacist." His nuclear family was filled with medical professionals. In addition to his parents, his brother Gérard became a gynecologist, with a career at Clinique Madeleine. Only his oldest brother, Jean-Marie, forged a different path, making his way as a geographer. Fayemi completed his high school studies in 1973, the year his mother died. A decade later, in 1983, he completed his pharmacy degree and married.[15]

Antonin Fayemi and his father Pierre illustrate the changes in the profession from the colonial to the postcolonial period. Even though Antonin was in the first generation of postcolonial pharmacists, a number of changes had already occurred. The most obvious improvement was that Antonin had greater autonomy in his professional practice. He was not required to commit a decade of his life to colonial service. Instead, soon after his graduation he began work at Laborex, a pharmaceutical wholesaler, with the approval of the National Order of Pharmacists.[16] He continued working there until he opened his own pharmacy.

Hélène Akindes

Francis d'Almeida and his daughter Hélène Akindes are another parent and child who practiced medicine in the colonial and postcolonial eras. Like Pierre Fayemi, Francis d'Almeida emigrated from Benin to Senegal; and like Antonin Fayemi, Hélène Akindes is Senegalese by birth. Her father was trained as a pharmacist and also worked at the Pasteur Institute. His work as a scientific analyst attracted the interest of his children. Akindes worked for many years in public pharmaceutical practice and in a laboratory before opening her pharmacy.[17]

Pape Amadou N'diaye

Pape N'diaye, who completed his degree in 1991, was one of many pharmacists interviewed who were born in, and worked solely in, postcolonial Senegal. The profession was much more liberalized when he joined it than it had been in previous generations. Pharmacy owners had much more freedom to choose their pharmacies' location, though they needed the approval of the National Order of Pharmacists. Moreover, when N'diaye opened his pharmacy in the 1990s, Senegal's pharmaceutical industry was engaging with new global partners. New drugs and technologies were becoming available, and existing ones were becoming cheaper. However, this younger generation of pharmacists also faced its own challenges, especially with deregulation. Many more students were admitted to the School of Pharmacy at the same time that laws restricting the number and location of pharmacies were relaxed. These changes presented a blessing and a curse. Some pharmacists were able to own pharmacies who would not have been able to otherwise, but the new policies allowed pharmacies to multiply in certain neighborhoods, competing fiercely for profits and clientele. As a result, some new pharmacies were destined to fail from the outset.

N'diaye was born in 1962 in the river basin of Senegal. He completed his primary education in Senegal and his secondary schooling in Mauritania, where his father worked. Like most Senegalese children, he also studied the Qur'an from a young age; he began at a Qur'anic school at age two. However, unlike many other students, he would continue this study until he was seventeen. He returned to his home country of Senegal in the 1980s to begin collegiate studies. He had originally planned to study medicine, but was told that he needed to wait to begin that program, so he decided to study pharmacy instead. He describes his study of pharmacy as an accident but finds the profession very rewarding.

When asked about the difficulties facing the profession, he emphasizes economic challenges. Inflation caused the costs of many pharmaceuticals and other supplies to increase, but not profits. The incomes of his customers have also remained stagnant. However, the most pressing difficulty he describes is pharmaceutical trafficking, which threatens public health. One popular street drug is *niebe*, "lion." This drug is a cortisteroid used to help women gain weight by retaining water. It is extremely dangerous, but is in demand because of social pressure on women to maintain a voluptuous figure.[18] N'diaye's reminisces confirm that pharmacists face challenges beyond professional interaction, development, and Western ideas of business management. Senegal's pervasive and elaborate formal and informal economic structures mean that Senegalese pharmacists face different challenges than do those in France.

N'deye Toutane Thiam Ngom

N'deye Toutane Ngom was born (in 1960) and raised in Dakar. She completed her secondary studies at Kennedy High School and began to study pharmacy. In her third year of pharmacy school, in 1984, she postponed her studies to accompany her husband to France. She returned to Senegal in 1987, and by 1990 she had completed her degree, the only member of her family to complete a pharmacy degree. She worked for several years in industry, with stints at a laboratory at Senegal's Pasteur Institute, before she was fortunate enough to receive a bank loan and an advance of products from a pharmaceutical wholesaler, which enabled her to open her own pharmacy.

Ngom had been drawn to the profession by fond memories of an older female cousin who had also studied pharmacy. Her cousin did not complete her studies, but her progress inspired Ngom nonetheless. When asked whether her children would follow her, Ngom responded, "I have a nephew who studied pharmacy until the third year and stopped. He was interested but began his study of biological studies too late. None of the others [i.e., her three sons] are interested. If I had a daughter, I think that she would be much more interested." Perhaps she thought a daughter would be drawn to the profession because of Ngom's own affinity for it and the prominence of women in the field. As a practicing pharmacist, she gained new sources of inspiration in addition to her cousin. She worked with

Khady Bao and cited N'deye Dieynaba Fall and Solange Decupper as role models.[19] All of these women were prominent pharmacists of the generation that followed Diop, Alcantara, and Fayemi.

Like Alcantara, who had opened his pharmacy five decades earlier, Ngom found that one of the greatest obstacles to succeeding as a pharmacy owner was the large influx of new pharmacy graduates each year. In fact, in the early 1990s the School of Pharmacy was graduating fewer than 150 pharmacy students a year. By the end of the century, this number had increased several-fold. Ngom argued that these graduates should go into a variety of fields: "We need to encourage those with pharmacy degrees to practice in other domains, such as biology, nutrition, environmental [development], homeopathic medicine, and industry, as contributions to the country."[20] This call is significant. Many of the pharmacists interviewed lamented the number of students graduating and of new pharmacies being opened. Their distress is understandable, as the profession is becoming saturated. Ngom moves beyond criticizing the situation to offer a potential solution.

Annette Seck N'diaye

Annette Seck N'diaye was born in 1961 to parents who had migrated to Dakar from the Casamance region of Senegal. Her heritage includes ancestors from Senegal, Portugal, and Guinea-Bissau. Both of her parents were educators. "My father was a professor of geography at the university and he wanted all of us to study medicine. We are three—one brother and two sisters. He wanted all of us to become doctors because it is a liberal profession. He also wanted us to open a clinic together."[21] His wishes were partially fulfilled, as all three siblings entered medical fields, each choosing a different specialization: she became a pharmacist, her brother a doctor, and her sister a dentist. Two of her cousins would later become pharmacists, and they spent their apprenticeships under her tutelage. Both became pharmacy owners in greater Dakar.

In the late twentieth century, N'diaye, Ngom, and Seck N'diaye were in their thirties and forties. Pharmacists of their generation were leaders and did not shy away from criticizing the expansion of the illegal pharmaceutical trade. They opened their pharmacies in lean economic times, when structural adjustment initiatives were being imposed, currency was being devalued, and infrastructure was disintegrating. They were able to use new developments in the profession, in shipping technologies, and in the internet to succeed in their businesses. They also would begin to diversify in creative new ways; Ngom and Seck N'diaye invested and served as consultants in other areas.

Shifting Demographics

During the first two decades of the postcolonial era, schools expanded and the number of students enrolled increased. Pharmacy programs were no exception, and as regulations regarding medical practice loosened, Senegalese began to gain a foothold as pharmacy owners. As the number of pharmacies owned by Senegalese nationals grew, so did the number of women who studied and practiced pharmacy. During the latter part of this period, women would gain prominence in the field. By the 1990s women owned the majority of pharmacies in Dakar.

Enrollment continued to increase at the School of Medicine and Pharmacy at Cheikh Anta Diop University through the latter part of the twentieth century, and the number of women pursuing higher education increased considerably. In 1967, 145 women and 1,336 men were enrolled in the School of Medicine and Pharmacy, and 3,630 women and 12,642 men were enrolled in Cheikh Anta Diop University as a whole; the proportion of female students thus ranged between 10 and 22 percent.[22] During the 1980s and 1990s, the number of pharmacy students rose dramatically: 696 students were enrolled in 1982–83, and 1,122 in 1987.[23] By the end of the century, about a thousand students were graduating in pharmacy each year. Further, during the 1983–84 school year, 52 percent of pharmacy students were women.[24] In 1991 and 1992, women made up a third of the entering students and almost 40 percent of graduating ones; 45 percent of entering female students went on to graduate.[25]

As their access to education improved, women began filtering into the medical professions, and some were studying and practicing pharmacy in Senegal as early as the 1940s and 1950s. Most of these pioneers were French, but some African women entered the field in these decades as well. Finding ways to navigate the formal economic sector and surmount obstacles such as gender and racial discrimination, they came to dominate the field by the end of the century. The next chapter will examine the flourishing of women pharmacists in postcolonial Senegal.

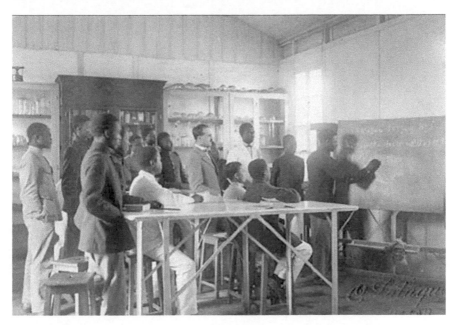

Training African pharmacists in Dakar, 1921. *Photograph courtesy of Archives d'Amicale Santé Navale et d'Outre Mer (ASNOM).*

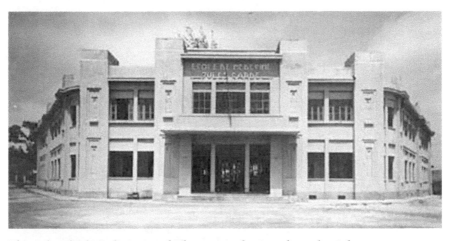

The School of Medicine and Pharmacy during the colonial era. *Photograph courtesy of Archives d'Amicale Santé Navale et d'Outre Mer (ASNOM).*

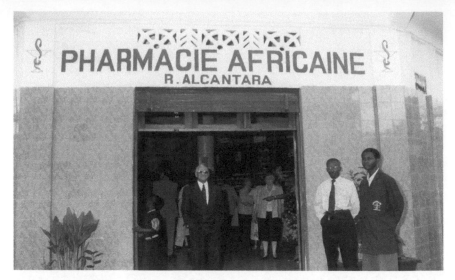

Pharmacie Africaine opened in 1949 and was owned by Rito Alcantara for more than fifty years. *Photograph in private collection.*

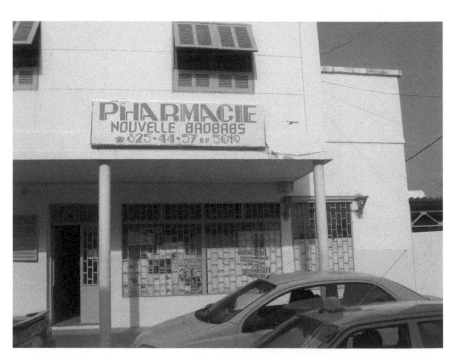

Pharmacie Nouvelle Baobabs, owned by Antonin Fayemi. *Photograph by Brahima Ouattara.*

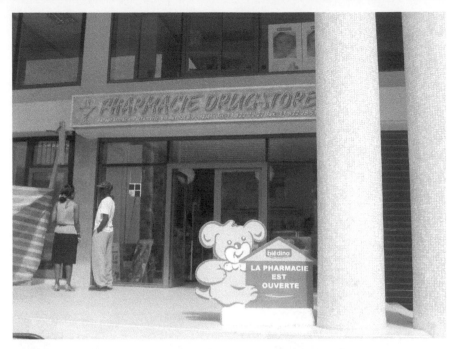

Pharmacie Drugstore opened in this location in 2008, after its earlier location was destroyed by fire. *Photograph by author.*

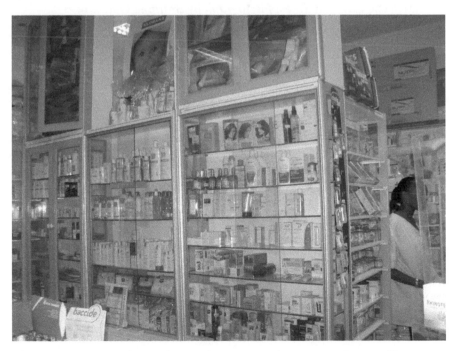

Pharmacie Pasteur, located near the Pasteur Institute and owned by N'deye Toutane Thiam Ngom. *Photograph by Brahima Ouattara.*

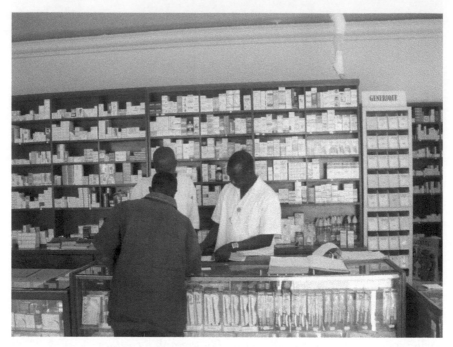

Dr. Alexandre Sylva and his assistant completing a customer transaction at Pharmacie Cayor in Thiès. *Photograph by Brahima Ouattara.*

3 Women Own Pharmacies Too: Financing Private Pharmacies

[Women] manage the household; they are there from beginning to end. Some women are hindered by tradition and other women face challenges after they marry but they manage their household. . . . If you give her an opening, a little training, some financial assistance, she can manage [any activity] very well.

—Aïssatou Moreau

"Where is the pharmacist?" asked a customer visiting Pharmacie Thiaroye-sur-Mer. "He will not return until the afternoon." "No, I want to speak to *her*." In the 1980s, exchanges similar to this one were common at Pharmacie Thiaroye-sur-Mer. Thérèze Gaye, the wife of François Gaye, often assisted him on the front lines of his pharmacy practice. Customers liked her, and some mistook her for a licensed pharmacist. By this time, many decades after Senegalese had first became pharmacy owners in the 1920s, local ideas about pharmacy had shifted. Women now worked as trained pharmacy assistants, and some owned pharmacies themselves. Many male pharmacists, in fact, hired women assistants to help with customers. The identity of a pharmacist became gendered as female in the local imagination, and women became synonymous with pharmacy.

Throughout the late colonial and early postcolonial periods, Senegalese women gained prominence in fields such as dentistry, medicine, and pharmacy. They became increasingly attracted to pharmacy, and by the late twentieth century, women owned 65 percent of the pharmacies in Dakar and 48 percent of those in Senegal. (Women pharmacists are mostly found in cities; few women own pharmacies in rural areas.) Research indicates this high proportion of female pharmacists is unique to Senegal. Women became more professionally active and used formal lending mechanisms to open private pharmacies. Their use of credit is significant in West Africa, where women have often had marginal access to diversified lines of credit.

This chapter examines how female pharmacists negotiated gender and professional development between 1945 and 2000. Above all, it explores how women used education and professional networks to gain prominence as pharmacy owners in Dakar. What led these women to become pharmacists? What obstacles did they face, and what strategies did they use to surmount these obstacles? This chapter also seeks to highlight the contribution of educated women by focusing on the experience of female pharmacy owners in greater Dakar. It considers how they have employed education, entrepreneurship, and professional networks to become prominent participants in the public health sector of Senegal.

Women's Economic Activity

Medical training in colonial (since 1918) and postcolonial Senegal represents the intersection of Western concepts of biomedical training with the realities of multifocal healing in local, predominately Muslim communities. Colonial authorities' decision to train more Africans in medicine, and the gradually increasing proportion of women among medical professionals, transformed notions of public health and social relations in the late colonial era. The creation of a large class of female pharmacists is an unanticipated and often overlooked legacy of the expansion of French biomedicine. When women began studying at the School of Medicine and Pharmacy in the 1940s and 1950s, it could not have been predicted that they would eventually create a professional class of educated women entrepreneurs who would transform societal notions of property ownership and familial relations. In the last decades of the twentieth century, as a result of their numbers and leadership, women became integral members of the pharmacy profession.

Scholarship has chronicled African women's economic activity in the informal and formal sectors. A large body of work investigates the employment of women in the informal sector.[1] Other studies explore their work as salaried professionals and as entrepreneurs in the formal sector.[2] Finally, several edited volumes include examples of women who work in the formal and informal sectors.[3] These studies examine a number of topics, including the intersections of colonial rule, education, and economics; professional networks; cultural transformations; social constraints; and familial obligations, especially in the colonial and postcolonial eras. Some scholars have specifically examined women's economic activity in Senegal, particularly that of women who earn their livelihood as religious healers, traders, and farmers.[4] The studies produced in the last four decades underscore the significance of women entrepreneurs to the economy of Senegal. However, most of them are not historical. Additionally, more work remains to be done on women who work in formal economies.

Few studies focus on female medical professionals in previously male-dominated industries. My study of female pharmacists and pharmacy owners is one of the first attempts to fill the vacuum in the field. This book extends earlier studies of African women, public health, and professionalization by examining how educated, professional women have created networks to improve their access to credit and their ability to open and run businesses. It also investigates the nuances of these women's lives as community members and caregivers. These multiple aspects of African women's lives mean that female pharmacists are active participants in Senegal's "economy of health."[5]

Women and Pharmacy Ownership

While scholars have published extensively on men's entrepreneurship in Francophone Africa, few have highlighted African women's entrepreneurial activity.[6] One exception is Fatou Sarr, who writes on entrepreneurial Senegalese women. In addition to commerce, she addresses the strategies women utilize to negotiate social and cultural spaces. Her work, however, does not provide a historical assessment of the intersection of gender and professional development in Senegal. Still, her analysis informs my unpacking of women pharmacists' professional and personal lives.

Women pharmacists are central to biomedical health care in Senegal, especially in Dakar, where many own their own businesses and offer many services in addition to the sale of medicine. Pharmacists are more numerous and certainly much more accessible to the public than are physicians in Senegal, thus they often diagnose and prescribe for the sick and ailing who come to their shops. They do not charge for consultations, and some even provide physicals and other examinations for their clients. Ill people often go to pharmacists before visiting medical doctors, because they cannot afford the higher prices that the latter charge for their time and treatments; many Senegalese turn to medical doctors only during emergencies, when circumstances compel them to visit clinics or hospitals. For these reasons, pharmacies occupy the forefront of health care in a nation with many other options, including a thriving indigenous health care system that includes both herbalists and Muslim healers, whose prayers and intercessions are valued in the predominately Muslim nation. In addition to conducting professional activities, these pharmacists—like most Senegalese women—manage domestic activities and negotiate gender roles in their extended families, their communities, and the broader society.

Women studied as midwives from the early colonial period. By 1928 they were training as nurses, and by the 1940s, they had begun studying and practicing pharmacy in Senegal. Pascale Barthélemy, who has published on midwives, argues that women's entry into these professional spheres helped "redefine women's social and familial roles."[7] Like Barthélemy, I am interested in the climate that helped to spur women's participation in professional spheres, particularly pharmacy. Looking at female pharmacists allows us to see how women entered professional fields with which they were not historically associated.

Most women who practiced pharmacy in the mid-twentieth century were French nationals who worked as assistants in established pharmacies. But in the 1940s, two French women, Mrs. Pétrau and Yvonne Chanteau, received the colonial authorities' approval to open pharmacies in Diourbel and Dakar, respectively.[8] Similarly, in 1950 Jacqueline Martin replaced Bernard Guigon, owner of Pharmacie Guigon, during his absence.[9] During this period, colonial policy capped the number of pharmacies in Dakar at twenty, and the number in Diourbel at only one. It is particularly noteworthy that the only pharmacy in Diourbel was female-owned.

During this period, African women were also starting to pursue medical studies. Between 1945 and 1952, two African women, Maïmouna Touré and Sara Coulibaly, graduated from the School of Medicine and Pharmacy.[10] Their names indicate that they were West African, perhaps Senegalese. Other women, such as Felicia N'diaye Basse, Maïmouna Soumah, and Marie Guéye, also practiced pharmacy during this period. Basse studied at the School of Medicine and Pharmacy in the late 1940s, but the records do not show her graduating; it is probable that she completed her degree abroad.[11] She owned and operated a pharmacy in Thiès, Pharmacie Cayor, for many years until her death in 2005. Soumah never opened a pharmacy but worked in the public health sector. According to N'deye Dieynaba Mbodj Fall, former president of the National Order of Pharmacists, Guéye did open a pharmacy.[12] However, I could find no record of her work in public or private archives. She has almost been erased from history.

Although these women were few, they are significant, because few people pursued advanced study in pharmacy during this period, and few of those who did were women. (Between the 1940s and the 1960s, female university enrollment was low; most women did not go beyond elementary school.) In 1945, four students were admitted to the pharmacy program at the School of Medicine and Pharmacy, thirty to the midwifery program, and forty-four to the medical program.[13] Two years later, in 1947, only forty pharmacists had received diplomas in French West Africa, compared to three hundred midwives and four hundred doctors. The few women pharmacists we have identified at that period thus constituted about 10 percent of all those practicing. In general, however, the gender divide among the medical professions was well defined. Pharmacy and medical graduates were almost all male, while midwives were women.

Several factors converged to allow women greater access to the medical professions. Women's access to education started to improve in French West Africa after independence. Female enrollment increased until women made up approximately 10 percent of matriculating students by 1969. In 1960, women were only 2 percent of the collegiate student population, but in 1968 they were 36 percent of the students at the School of Medicine and Pharmacy, and by the late 1970s that proportion had reached 52 percent. This growth in the number of women studying pharmacy coincided with the increase in the number of women college enrollees between 1967 and 1991.[14]

Undoubtedly, women faced discrimination at the School of Medicine and Pharmacy, and a number of those who graduated in the first wave of female professionalization spoke of it. An unspoken rule ensured that a smaller proportion of qualified women than qualified men were admitted to the pharmacy program.[15] Despite this discrimination, women showed tenacity and commitment; often they made up a higher proportion of a class upon graduation than they had in their first year.

In addition, the increase in the number of French female pharmacy owners and medical administrators may have benefited African women. It was becoming more acceptable for women to play a variety of roles in the public health sector. In fact, in 1961, a female French pharmacist, Françoise Gobert Marcelle, was appointed director of one of Senegal's pharmacy companies.[16] In the following decade Solange Decupper, a Senegalese woman, became head of the Syndicate of Private Senegalese Pharmacists, or Pharmacy Syndicate, a powerful professional organization for pharmacists in private practice. Samir Amin finds that only ten Africans owned pharmacies in the region between Dakar and Thiès at this period.[17] It is evident that at least two of them, Solange Decupper and Felicia N'diaye Basse, were women.

In the 1960s, Senegalese women rapidly gained prominence in pharmacy. During the 1970s and 1980s, they became the face of pharmacy ownership in Senegal. This is particularly significant in a country where, as late as the 1940s and 1950s, many African professionals faced racial discrimination. African women faced double discrimination, on the grounds of both race and gender. In addition to surmounting these barriers, female pharmacists also transformed how women navigated the formal economy.

Decupper opened a pharmacy in 1966. She was among the most respected of the practicing pharmacists I interviewed. Many younger pharmacists sought internships with her, and older ones often described her as the foremost female pharmacy owner in Senegal. Official records and interviews suggest that she was the first black person to open a pharmacy in the downtown area.[18] Although Senegal had been independent since 1960, there was still an enormous French presence in the capital; about 20 percent of Dakar's population was French.[19] Many of the French expatriates still owned pharmacies, and the early postcolonial years were filled with significant professional negotiations. Decupper opened her pharmacy during this transitional period in Senegal's history.

She named her business Pharmacie Drugstore because she wanted to model it after pharmacies in the United States. She tried to situate it in an American-style shopping center and maintain American-style business hours. Senegalese pharmacies normally closed for a siesta in the middle of the day, and often closed for the day in early evening. Decupper decided that she would only close her pharmacy for a short afternoon break, and afterward stay open until midnight. This policy was revolutionary, and it threw her into conflict with established pharmacists.[20]

Not only had this Senegalese woman been able to secure a prime location, she now wanted to change established ways of doing business. Decupper explained that she wanted to honor the demands of the population and be more accessible to her clientele. She admitted that her decision created a great deal of tension, saying that "the French made war" on her, but argued, "No law prevented this change." She found an ally in François Gaye, then president of the Pharmacy Syndicate. He acted as an intermediary between Decupper and other downtown pharmacists, some of whom gradually realized the economic benefits of her policy and later followed her lead. The location of Decupper's pharmacy and her business success made her one of Senegal's most prominent pharmacists, which enabled her to represent not only the interests of Senegal's pharmacy owners but also those of emerging female pharmacists. She was both an advocate and a role model for many of the female pharmacists who emerged between the 1970s and 1990s.

Gaining Influence: Women as Prominent Office Holders

Decupper's story illustrates the transformations brewing in early postcolonial Senegal. From the mid-1960s through the mid-1980s, more and more French nationals left the country, and the postcolonial Senegalese state instituted a series of new policies. The administration of President Léopold Senghor hoped to "Africanize" several professional classes, including the medical educational sector. Over almost the next twenty years, the state pursued this policy by supporting existing medical professionals, offering business loans, and expanding access to education at all levels from primary school to university. These transformations of the political and social climate created a professional opening in which female pharmacists could maneuver. Many women who completed pharmacy studies in the 1960s and 1970s in Senegal were able to capitalize on these developments to obtain leadership positions.

Several women gained prominence and held professional office in the 1970s in the field of pharmacy, of whom the most prominent were Solange Decupper and N'deye Dieynaba Mbodj Fall.[21] From 1974 to 1994, Decupper served as the president of the Pharmacy Syndicate. In this position, she represented private pharmacy owners and was a liaison between them, the government, local and foreign pharmacy suppliers and drug manufacturers, and consumers. The office of the Pharmacy Syndicate is most concerned with the entrepreneurial aspects of running a pharmacy: economic viability, promotion of business, and market dominance. This position of influence allowed Decupper to represent not only the interests of Senegal's pharmacy owners but also those of emerging female pharmacists. Several female pharmacists spoke of Decupper's direct and indirect influence on their professional lives, speaking of her as a mentor and role model. Indeed, a significant number of informants, old and young, male and female, saw her as the embodiment of female pharmacy ownership in Senegal. One pharmacist, Marie Emilienne Tavares, who received post-graduate training under Decupper's tutelage, warmly described her as a good mentor.[22]

On 19 January 1975, N'deye Dieynaba Mbodj Fall was elected president of the National Order of Pharmacists in the second round of votes, defeating two men: Rito Alcantara and Moustapha Kandji.[23] In this position, which she held for more than two decades, Fall was the most powerful pharmacist in the country. The National Order of Pharmacists is an umbrella organization that encompasses most pharmacy associations in Senegal. It has both public and private administrative divisions and includes the Union of Young Senegalese Pharmacists and the professors of pharmacy at the School of Medicine and Pharmacy.

During the long period in which she served her profession, Fall oversaw the creation of hundreds of new pharmacies, corresponded with officials of the Senegalese Ministry of Health and with private pharmaceutical companies (mostly French, but also those of other countries), managed professional conflicts, and lobbied the Senegalese state on educational matters, drug regulations, and the illegal underground trade in pharmaceuticals. As a result, she and her board had extensive power. Senegal's law no. 73-62 of 19 December 1962, establishing the National Order of Pharmacists (Ordre national des pharmaciens), dictates that people wishing to own a pharmacy must hold a degree in pharmacy and must describe their background, education, and experience, as well as agreeing to uphold professional guidelines. However, merely being qualified to own a pharmacy is no guarantee of actually being able to do so. Since the 1980s, in particular, the number of pharmacy students has ballooned, and not all who want to open pharmacies will be granted the right. The National Order of Pharmacists determines which requests are granted and approves or vetoes the location of the proposed pharmacy. While many women and men became pharmacy owners during Fall's term as president, opening pharmacies soon after their graduation, others did not fare as well; many were not able to do so until several years after earning their degrees.

As women became more numerous in the profession, others came to hold leadership positions. Anta Sar, owner of Pharmacie Mermoz, recalls, "Even in the associations . . . at the level of the [National] Order [of Pharmacists] and the [Pharmacy] Syndicate, women were involved for a long time. The leaders of the Order and the Syndicate have both been women. Women were the majority, and they worked hard and they fought for their dignity to occupy their place in society."[24] From 1983 to 1999, Khady Bao was the president of Council Section B, the arm of the National Order of Pharmacists representing those in private practice, and between 1998 and 2000 other women, including Maïmouna Diop, N'deye Toutane Thiam Ngom, and Annette Seck N'diaye, also held leadership positions. In 1999, Diop replaced Bao as president of Council Section B, a position she held for four years; she had previously been secretary general of the Pharmacy Syndicate. Ngom was the treasurer of the National Order of Pharmacists and very active at the headquarters of the organization, and Annette Seck N'diaye became president of the Pharmacy Syndicate.[25] Diop, Seck N'diaye, and Ngom collaborated with their male colleagues to organize an international pharmaceutical forum in 2001. After Fall resigned as the president of the National Order of Pharmacists in 1999, she was replaced by a man; the president of Council Section A (representing public pharmacists, such as state bureaucrats and university professors) was also a man. Nonetheless, women remained visible in leadership positions. Like the female leaders before them, they continued to consolidate their power.

Born in 1944 in Saint-Louis, Khady Kebe Bao married a biomedical physician, received her degree in 1973, and opened her pharmacy in 1974 with the assistance of loans of 6 million CFA francs from a bank and 12 million from a pharmaceutical supplier. Bao's pharmacy, Du Guet, was situated in the downtown district of Dakar and was quite lucrative for many years. Bao was very active in many of the professional organizations, including serving as president of Council Section B, the commercial arm of the Pharmacy Syndicate, during the mid-1990s, and she influenced a number of younger women.

Eventually, however, the pharmacy's profit margins fell; she grossed between 20 and 30 million CFA francs per year in the mid-1990s, very low considering her excellent location. She blamed this poor performance on the rapid, unregulated proliferation of pharmacies, which she compared to "the expansion of telephone booths." Because of this, she decided to sell her business. Her children were now adults, and she did not have the economic responsibilities that many other pharmacists did, so the decision was easier for her than it would have been for others. In 1998 she sold her pharmacy to Mohamed Ghandour for 70 million CFA francs, including 7 million for the business name, 9.3 million for official materials, and 25.7 million for stock.[26]

Her daughter, Nafissatou "Nafi" Mbaye, was attracted to pharmacy because of her mother's involvement in the field. In 1993, a few years after completing her graduate work (which she, unlike her mother, did in France),[27] she opened Pharmacie Darabis on Bourguiba Avenue, a major thoroughfare. While the proliferation of pharmacies hurt the profitability of her mother's pharmacy, Mbaye's clientele was growing. Her pharmacy was located in a fairly moderate neighborhood known as Sicap Darabis, to which people came regularly to shop, study, and catch public transportation. It also received a steady flow of foreigners, who often visited her pharmacy. The adjacent neighborhood, Grand Dakar, is economically diverse but generally less wealthy than Sicap Darabis. Since Pharmacie Darabis opened, however, the community has grown considerably. Consequently, the location of her pharmacy allows her to attract a diverse group of regular clients. Like her mother, Mbaye recognizes the importance of professional alliances and has been a major player in her generation of pharmacists. During my interviews with her, she said that marketing and consistent working hours had been central to her success in business.[28]

One of my more noteworthy findings is that so many daughters and granddaughters of pharmacists also became pharmacists. Some chose the profession themselves, while many had the decision made for them by a parent or other senior family member. For example, Bineta Dia's father chose her career. Her family included two doctors, and her mother was a midwife.[29] Two other pharmacists of this generation emphasized the influence of their parents. Hawoly Sy credited her father, Abdoul Birane Wane, with attracting her to the field: "My father was a pharmacist; I wanted to be like him." Indeed, she named her pharmacy Abdoul Birane, after him.[30] Her professional career overlapped for a few years with her father's, as Mbaye's did with her mother's. After retiring, Abdoul Wane sold his pharmacy to Aby Kane Diallo.[31] Many others who opened pharmacies in the 1980s and 1990s had at least one relative who worked in the health sector.

Family influence is one of the reasons that pharmacy ownership has burgeoned during the past two decades. Another is the changes, in 1981, to the laws regulating the density of pharmacies. In 1986, there were 72 pharmacies in Dakar and 109 in Senegal. In 1994, there were 116 in Dakar and 240 in Senegal.[32] As of 2000, there were 240 pharmacies in Dakar and 517 in Senegal. The number of Dakar pharmacies thus doubled in less than ten years. During the course of my research, a new pharmacy opened near my home and I was informed of several others.

Most respondents criticized the rapid expansion of pharmacies, yet many probably would not have been able to own one if the law had not changed. The 1981 legislation increased the allowable density from one pharmacy for every fifteen thousand people to one for every ten thousand, and established criteria for how close they could be to one another in densely populated areas.[33] Since the 1990s, the School of Pharmacy has produced approximately a hundred graduates every year. Most will never have the option of opening their own pharmacies in such a saturated market.

Funding Pharmacies

Much of the literature on women and development represents women as victims because of their limited access to credit and property.[34] The existing scholarship suggests that women gain access to credit primarily through informal mechanisms, such as the rotating credit associations found in many African societies.[35] In contrast, Senegal's women pharmacists tell another story. Owning a pharmacy is a major enterprise in Senegal. The pharmacist often owns the building, the land it rests on, and the stock and equipment inside. Female pharmacists not only have more access to credit than the literature might suggest, they are also simultaneously medical professionals, property owners, employers, and managers. The women interviewed for this project acquired capital for their pharmacies in a variety of ways, including petitioning formal lending societies, drawing on personal savings, and receiving gifts from family members. Many used loans from banks, pharmaceutical companies, the government, and wholesale companies to pay some portion of their start-up costs. While not all pharmacists take out loans, many of them benefit from their availability.

The female pharmacists I interviewed gave a variety of reasons for their access to credit. Some said that they could get loans because they had degrees. But many Senegalese hold diplomas yet are ineligible for financial assistance. Their choice of profession is a more important factor. Pharmacists are trusted members of the community who often create and maintain lucrative enterprises. Moreover, their work is performed in public, making it difficult for them to avoid paying back loans. In general, their social position, capital investment, and career choice allow them to gain access to credit networks unavailable to most women entrepreneurs.

Despite the fact that many of these women did not own land or a house prior to opening a pharmacy, they were still able to get credit. About half the pharmacists interviewed relied completely or partially on a bank loan to finance their pharmacy. Another significant portion took loans from pharmaceutical manufacturers or wholesalers in order to buy initial stock, while others relied on personal savings. Dozens of informants reported relying on formal lending agencies at some point in their career. Only a few pharmacists mentioned difficulties in getting bank loans.

Marième N'diaye did not even need one; she was able to open her pharmacy with a combination of personal savings and familial support.[36] Others, such as Maïmouna Diop and Marie Emilienne Tavares, relied on a combination of savings and loans. Diop, owner of Pharmacie Limaloulaye, was one of the early pharmacists in the suburb of Guediawaye, on the outskirts of metropolitan Dakar. She recalled,

> I do not think that women are discriminated against with access to credit. If a woman meets all of the conditions of a man then she should have equivalent access. I started modestly. I had worked in the pharmaceutical industry and saved my salary to contribute to my pharmacy. It was not as easy to get credit as it is now, and I took a loan of one million CFA from a bank. I did, however, also rely on loans from wholesalers [to stock her pharmacy].[37]

Similarly, Tavares, owner of Pharmacie Cephas, worked in the industry for fifteen years before opening her pharmacy; she was unmarried and had owned her pharmacy for two years when she was interviewed. She found the early years of pharmacy ownership challenging but cited the success of her mentors, including Decupper, as motivation to continue. Like Seck N'diaye, Tavares also took a loan from a bank to start out and had recently finished repaying it at the time of her first interview. "I tightened the belt and did not eat anything in order to reimburse the bank."[38] All of these women had different experiences opening their pharmacies, but their comments illustrate their access to formal lending mechanisms.

In the latter half of the twentieth century, the numbers of women in pharmacy grew exponentially. As women became officeholders in professional organizations, they created new power networks from which to assist new female pharmacists. Despite the challenges of governmental regulation as well as domestic and international economic crises, they capitalized on their education, business acumen, and local and global professional networks to become prominent members of Senegal's health care sector. Because they were professionals and business owners, they had more autonomy than their female counterparts who worked in other sectors. They have had access to both formal and informal sectors and have been forerunners in a previously male-dominated profession. As the respondents illustrate, in less than four decades Senegalese women not only integrated the previously male-dominated industry but transformed it. The narratives and business records of women like Bao, Decupper, and Moreau show that women not only studied pharmacy and pursued entrepreneurial opportunities, but were also formidable participants in economic life. Owning pharmacies with a consistent consumer base, women have emerged as the face of biomedical care in Senegal.

4   House and Street: Negotiating Professional and Private Lives

I am not a feminist but I think that women's roles are very important. Women are everywhere. They are mothers and are found in every profession. They fight for respect.

—Maïmouna N'diaye Niang

In the postcolonial period, it became easier to open a pharmacy, and the number of pharmacies in Senegal rose rapidly. By 1994, 80 percent of all pharmaceutical sales in Senegal were made by privately owned pharmacies. Pharmacies were attractive to customers because they were well stocked and professionally managed. But despite these advances in the field, pharmacists who owned private pharmacies faced a number of challenges. Women pharmacists, especially, had to balance the demands of family and work in a predominately Muslim society that had preconceived notions about women and labor. All pharmacists, regardless of their gender, also faced economic challenges during this period.

Pharmacy owners were keen entrepreneurs who contributed to public health and participated in professional networks. They tried to earn a reasonable profit, which became increasingly difficult over the course of the late twentieth century, as currency devaluations and other aspects of externally mandated structural adjustment policies

(SAPs) disrupted businesses dependent upon imports. This chapter explores Senegalese pharmacists' professional and private lives and how they responded to these social and economic challenges in the changing local and global terrain. In doing so, it contributes new ideas to the existing scholarship on the management of family and work in African history.

Negotiating Social and Familial Demands

Since the late 1960s, Senegal's pharmacists have been a diverse group with various ethnic and religious backgrounds, reflecting the cultural breadth of Senegalese society. Most have been Muslim, with a smaller percentage of Catholics, and most have been married. Many had at least one Wolof parent.[1] Some had mixed racial or national origins, with roots in Morocco, Cape Verde, France, or Guinea, and became Senegalese through naturalization or marriage.

Regardless of ethnic and religious background, Senegalese society considers women to be mothers and nurturers before all else. They are expected to bear children, manage household logistics, and maintain relationships with neighbors and extended family. Female pharmacists and pharmacy students were not exempt from these expectations. A significant number of the female pharmacists interviewed for this study pursued their studies while balancing the responsibilities of a husband and children.[2] The interviewed women averaged three or four children, but some, such as Marie Emilienne Bâ, owner of Pharmacie Cheikh Amadou Bamba, had many more. She gave birth to eight children during the course of her studies and the early years of managing her pharmacy.[3]

Women of all educational backgrounds are expected to be active in family life. Even when they hire domestic help, all women—wives, mothers, and female members of the extended family—are expected to contribute to the interworkings of the familial base. It is still more acceptable for a male pharmacist to spend long hours at work, without arranging for a surrogate caregiver or being engaged with the nuances of home life.

In response to socially based gender expectations, female pharmacists developed strategies to negotiate social and familial demands while also maintaining their professional careers. One female pharmacist, Hawoly Wane Sy, owned a pharmacy at the fringes of Dakar's commercial center, but she lived in the middle-class neighborhood of Point E. The distance between them meant that she faced a long commute each day. She spoke about the concessions that women are required to make to simultaneously manage professional and familial spheres: "Owning a pharmacy is difficult for the family. My pharmacy closes at 8:30 PM, and sometimes I am required to stay [at work] until midnight. I am looking to hire someone who can relieve me during the evening."[4] Several women emphasized their long commutes, because they further reduced the time spent at home. Male pharmacists did not mention the challenges of commuting in their interviews.

A number of pharmacists similarly spoke of the possibility of hiring a trained assistant to relieve the pressure of work and allow them to better accommodate their family and work commitments. Some other women sought the support of female family members or maids to assist with domestic chores. In fact, many middle-class and elite Senegalese women—not just pharmacists—hire one or more domestic workers to help with meal preparation, child and elder care, shopping, and other responsibilities. Most domestic servants live with their employers from Monday through Saturday, making them available both day and night. Touty Diack Dia, owner of Pharmacie Thiaroye-sur-Mer, explained, "I have an assistant, and this allows me to complete several different tasks. I work a continuous day between 8:00 AM and 3:30 PM and devote the afternoons to my family. Obviously, this creates some tension with my clientele. Generally, it is during the afternoon that many of them leave work and come [to the pharmacy] for counsel, but I must take care of my family."[5] Khady Bengeloum Diallo, owner of Pharmacie Zahra, also addressed this issue: "In the beginning, it was difficult. I opened the pharmacy at 8:00 AM and it closed at midnight. In this environment, one must have a husband who is very understanding. Now, things have changed; I generally do not work beyond the afternoon. I now guard this time for my family."[6] These stories provide a living record of the ways in which female pharmacists strategically juggle their professional and personal commitments.

Annette Seck N'diaye also spoke about this issue. Seck N'diaye, who was president of the Pharmacy Syndicate from 1999 to 2003, suggested that gender-specific constraints pushed women into owning pharmacies rather than working for others. She noted, stating the first sentence in English for emphasis, that when "you work for yourself, you do not face as many problems." She argued that women faced widespread gender discrimination in industry. If a woman works for a drug manufacturer, for example, production cannot stop to accommodate childbirth and a three- to four-month period of recuperation. As a result, a woman's job is in jeopardy if she is required to answer to others. "If they have a choice between hiring a man or a woman—men will receive more consideration. It is a question of profit margins."[7] These comments demonstrate that women pharmacists have a keen understanding of the cultural considerations and social constraints they face as female professionals.

Other seasoned pharmacists, including Mariane Coly and Solange Decupper, also spoke of the negotiations that professional women undertake to maintain societal standards. Coly was in her sixties when interviewed for this project. Raised as a Catholic in a Wolof family from Rufisque, she became a pharmacist following the direction and guidance of her father. Indeed, men were her earliest examples of pharmacists. She received her diploma in 1970 and bought her store, Pharmacie du Théâtre, in downtown Dakar in 1976 with a bank loan. Like many of her colleagues, she valued interaction with clients as an essential aspect of her profession. Nonetheless, she contended that running a pharmacy is harder for women than for men because after the work day is over women have more responsibilities in taking care of children (she had four with her businessman husband) and little opportunity for rest.[8] Decupper agreed, saying, "Black women are superwomen. Women manage their profession, homes, children as well as other commitments. 'Bravo, la femme

noire—c'est vraiment un superwoman'" ["Bravo, the black woman—
she is truly a superwoman"].[9]

Anta Sar takes a slightly different approach to balancing the demands of work and family than the other women. She agrees that it
is challenging, especially since she has daughters, but argues that her
professional life takes precedence. Since she lives in the same building her pharmacy is in, she does not face the problem of a long commute, but still says, "Between the two, pharmacy and home, I work all
the time. I open the pharmacy very early in the morning. I do have a
[pharmacy] assistant and we work well together. My mother, my sisters, and a housekeeper are also available to help with my home duties. When my professional duties require my presence, I prefer to
choose my profession. My husband is very understanding. He runs
errands for me in the evenings, such as going to the bank."[10] Dr. Sar's
approach to her business clearly indicates the multiple avenues open
to these educated, professional women. She works long hours but
maintains a family-work balance through the support of female and
male family members. Since her pharmacy and home are in the same
building, she is able to closely manage activities in both domains. By
drawing on a variety of resources, women pharmacists translate and
navigate between differing cultural beliefs, ideas about healing systems, and notions of gender in their quest for professional success.

Women pharmacists have pioneered new ideas about the roles
women hold in Senegalese society. Scholars Elisabeth McMahon and
Corrie Decker have illustrated how societal ideas about women's respectability influence a woman's professional life in East Africa.[11]
While Senegal has its own ideas of respectability, Senegalese society
generally expects working women to maintain a respectable household presence. They can do so with their own labor or the labor of
others, as we have seen.

While not all family members may welcome the hours that women
pharmacists work, many were impressed with the potential economic
benefits of having a successful pharmacist in their family. Often some
members of their immediate or, more frequently, extended family expected the women to contribute financially to official and unofficial

holidays, celebrations, and family milestones such as marriages, funerals, burials, pilgrimages, baptisms, and celebrations of Tabaski, Korité, and Ramadan.[12] Aïssatou Moreau, owner of Pharmacie Chifaoun, spoke of these familial expectations: "Women spend considerable time regulating certain problems, which in some cases may lead to a problem with record keeping. There are times when these women . . . are required to spend money . . . for exaggerated expenses such as baptisms, marriages, and trips to Mecca. There are other social pressures after you start working."[13] Attendees at these types of social events often include neighbors, friends, and acquaintances in addition to immediate and extended family members. From a few dozen to several hundred people may visit and eat at the home on a single day. Accordingly, the monetary and social costs of these events can be quite significant. While many of the female pharmacists interviewed were committed to assisting with these events, they also spoke of the economic burden doing so could create.

In Senegalese society, the power to make major decisions affecting the extended family has usually been reserved to elders, usually male. But the economic status of these female pharmacists has been transformative, giving them the power to affect such decisions when they feel it appropriate.

Motherhood and marriage are among the most important aspects of Senegalese women's lives. Women's narratives of marriage and motherhood are found in oral histories and semiautobiographical novels.[14] These primary and secondary accounts of women's experiences help to illuminate their social obligations. In Senegal, as in many other African countries, women respond to social constructions of motherhood, marriage, and the pursuit of a career. Wifehood and motherhood can take on multiple configurations.

While a few of the female pharmacists who participated in this project were divorced, most were married. Furthermore, most of the married women were in first marriages; only a few had divorced (or been widowed) and remarried. In Africa, as in most of the world, women who divorce their spouses tend to have been more financially independent during their marriages than other married women. The few divorced women I spoke with seemed secure in their status and in some cases remained unmarried indefinitely. Their financial security enabled them to support themselves and their children.[15] Official counts of divorced women in Senegal are generally low and do not take into consideration the fact that many divorced women quickly remarry. "Marriage is more much flexible among Muslims than among Christians. . . . While the Qur'an limits the numbers of wives a polygamous man may have, it does not define how many times one can marry and divorce during a lifetime, thereby allowing great flexibility in unions."[16] Since polygyny is pervasive in Senegal, it is significant to the ways pharmacy owners balance family and work. Interviewees were not asked if they were in polygynous unions, and none said they were; but even if none of my informants are polygynously married, they have parents, siblings, and extended family members who are. Some were the children of polygynous unions. Both nuclear and extended families in Senegal are extremely cohesive. Thus, polygyny can impact larger family decisions, including about the family celebrations to which pharmacy owners often contribute.[17]

The women quoted above identify ways they negotiate the demands of family and work. Their comments illuminate the negotiations made by many women pharmacists. To be sure, these women are able to hire pharmacy assistants, because their pharmacies are sufficiently profitable. Other pharmacists with less lucrative pharmacies are not able to pursue such options. Many of the owners who own less profitable enterprises work longer hours and hire office managers or unofficial pharmacy assistants. Unofficial assistants are not trained in pharmacy, but the pharmacist may train them in the basics.

Pharmacy Ownership: Constraints and Success

While familial considerations loom large in the lives of all professional women and men, pharmacy owners confront a host of distinct challenges. Some are local, some regional, and some originate outside the African continent. The pharmacy profession is highly regulated. Changes in the economic environment, a rise in global health insecurity, and new transnational intersections have forced pharmacists to respond to these challenges in flexible and innovative ways. Doing so requires business acumen and an understanding of this changing global marketplace.

Some aspects of postcolonial pharmacy regulation were inherited from the colonial era, and others were new initiatives by the independent Senegalese state. Some colonial regulations were adapted and used as models for policy in the postcolonial era, including requirements for owning a pharmacy, standards of professional conduct, and strict guidelines for staffing. Others, such as required distances between pharmacies and increased rigor in pharmaceutical training, were new in the postcolonial era. While health policy is approved by the Senegalese Ministry of Health, pharmaceutical associations—especially the National Order of Pharmacists—have also greatly influenced pharmacy practice.

The National Order of Pharmacists was created in 1962 and has been one of Senegal's most prominent professional associations.[18] In the same year, the Senghor cabinet issued a document that laid the framework for this new organization by describing its goals and membership requirements. Article 2 stated that pharmacists could not practice their profession in Senegal without being members of the National Order of Pharmacists.[19] The only exceptions to this rule were Senegalese or foreign pharmacists who were in active military service. Council Section A of the National Order of Pharmacists included "public pharmacists" (e.g., state bureaucrats, university professors, and others) who did not practice pharmacy for profit, unlike pharmacists in Section B.

During this early post-independence period, the Senegalese government continued to direct resources to the public health sector, which was governed by the Ministry of Health. As part of the president's cabinet, the minister of health often had direct access to the president and the prime minister. Another administrative department, the Directorate of Pharmacy, was the most active regulator of pharmacy policy. Its personnel oversaw the writing, revision, and enforcement of relevant laws. Pharmacists employed by the Directorate of Pharmacy were classified as part of Section A in the National Order of Pharmacists.

The pharmacists I surveyed own their own pharmacies, and are thus classified as members of Section B. Many of them are also members of the Pharmacy Syndicate and other, smaller organizations. In general, many of the pharmacists in Section B have higher incomes, more autonomy, and more flexible work schedules than those in Section A.

Some countries, such as Ethiopia, have limited the number and autonomy of privately owned pharmacies in favor of government-run establishments.[20] Despite these policies, privately owned pharmacies in Ethiopia, like those in Senegal, are concentrated in densely populated urban neighborhoods, and rural populations have limited access to them. In fact, in Senegal, government-run medical supply depots are prominent in rural areas, whereas in Ethiopia the inequities between rural and urban health care are more apparent. This is particularly concerning because 85 percent of Ethiopia's population lives in rural areas, compared to 50 percent in Senegal.

While the laws governing the number and spacing of pharmacies in Senegal are quite generous, the qualifications for opening and owning a pharmacy are strictly regulated. No one can open a pharmacy who has not studied pharmacy, earned a pharmacy license, and studied under an established pharmacist for three months. However, pharmacists can hire other people to practice in their pharmacies. Those applying to open a pharmacy must provide a birth certificate, a copy of their diploma, a survey of the neighborhood they intend to open in, and a blueprint of the planned pharmacy, and must submit requests to the National Order of Pharmacists and the Ministry of Health.[21] Even successfully submitting all of these documents and acquiring funding does not secure pharmacy ownership; factors such as population density, zoning, and politics also play a role in the process.

Like pharmacists who own pharmacies, pharmacists working in industry are also subject to government oversight through the Ministry of Health. Furthermore, the National Order of Pharmacists also regulates this professional trajectory. In 1985, a Dr. Touré sent a memo to both the National Order of Pharmacists and the Ministry of Health requesting permission to work as a pharmacist for Parke Davis.[22] In 1983, Antonin Fayemi submitted a similar request to be allowed to work at Laborex.[23] High-ranking members of the National Order of Pharmacists, in some cases, wielded as much power as the Ministry of Health in regulating aspects of private pharmacy practice and pharmaceutical policy.

Despite the strength of their authority, the National Order of Pharmacists has gradually made concessions during the postcolonial era to respond to the widespread desire to own a pharmacy. While the majority of pharmacy graduates did not go into private practice, the number who did began to increase significantly. For decades, pharmacies were not constructed near hospitals and major clinics. By the late 1980s, this regulation was loosened and Pharmacie Nelson Mandela was built directly across from the Hôpital Principal, the biggest public hospital in the country. Similarly, Pharmacie Pasteur was built almost directly across the street from the Pasteur Institute. The Pasteur Institute caters to a different and smaller clientele than the Hôpital Principal, but a number of pharmacy owners objected to the location of both of these pharmacies. The pharmacy associations and the Directorate of Pharmacy were not always effective at reducing competition. One of the ways that the leadership responded was by frequently revising the required distance between pharmacies or the permitted density of pharmacies per capita, to try to contain their numbers.

Economic Flux and the Devaluation of Currency

As a more robust pharmacy network emerged in the postcolonial era, it confronted economic concerns from both within and beyond the Senegalese state, with important consequences for Senegalese pharmacists. After the French government transferred power in 1960, Senegal moved into independence with one of the most developed economies in West Africa. In addition to substantial infrastructure and health and educational services, Senegal had a highly profitable agricultural export economy based primarily on peanuts. By the mid-1970s, however, the peanut market had become increasingly dependent on global market fluctuations.

From 1964 to 1975, the government spent large sums to create industrial zones and finance industrial expansion. Large percentages of the annual budget also went to social projects. The government spent more than it could take in, however, and increasingly relied on international donors for survival. Gradually, the International Monetary Fund and the World Bank began to impose structural adjustment programs (SAPs). In the 1980s and 1990s, Senegal implemented several SAPs, with varying success. In addition to support from the IMF and the World Bank, Senegal received loans and grants from a variety of sources including the European Union, USAID, and the governments of Saudi Arabia and Kuwait.[24]

One of the most radical economic shocks was the devaluation of the local currency, the CFA franc, by 50 percent on 12 January 1994. The devaluation was intended to promote exports and attract tourists, but it did not dramatically bolster the local economy. Exports were still hindered by tariffs, and some markets, like the United States, would not fully open up for several more years. Tourism improved somewhat. Overall, these economic reforms negatively affected local and national government budgets and entrepreneurs and created a significant financial burden for millions of Francophone Africans.

In particular, the currency devaluation doubled debt burdens and reduced consumer buying power, which affected pharmacists. The president of the National Order of Pharmacists, N'deye Dieynaba Fall, responded to the crisis on 25 March with a memo to her colleagues. In it she emphasized the consequences of this fiscal policy for private pharmacies, which primarily traded in imported goods. She called for pharmacists to meet and discuss how to approach this major challenge amongst themselves and in tandem with government officials.[25] As president, she effectively lobbied elected officials about the needs of private pharmacy owners.

Most importantly for the industry, this reduction in buying power decreased the disposable income of pharmacy clients and prompted increasing numbers of them to try to save money by buying biomedical pharmaceuticals from parallel (black) pharmaceutical markets. At the same time, the loans that pharmacy owners had taken out to buy property, stock, and other items had now doubled in value. Pharmacy owners therefore had to increase the prices of their stock to offset these new economic demands. Because these changes happened rapidly, a large percentage of the Senegalese population was unable to cope well with the major economic recession. Finally, many of the investors in the parallel market noticed these changing dynamics and chose to capitalize on market conditions.

During interviews for this project, informants were asked about the difficulties of pharmacy ownership, but the devaluation was not specifically mentioned. Nonetheless, many informants commented frequently on it, as well as on the proliferation of pharmacies and growth of the parallel trade. Among them were Mame Awa Guèye Diop, owner of Pharmacie Lat Dior, and Marie Emilienne Bâ, owner of Pharmacie Cheikh Amadou Bamba. Bâ lamented the devaluation and said that it caused prices to increase for pharmacists and clients alike.[26]

A Financial Picture of Pharmacy Ownership

Despite these challenges, many of Senegal's privately owned pharmacies have been profitable in the postcolonial period, underscoring their significance to the public health care sector. One way of measuring their success is to count the number of pharmacy assistants (PAs) employed in the industry in Dakar. PAs must have received formal training in pharmacy; they are often new pharmacy graduates or pharmacists who were unable to find the capital to open their own pharmacies. Between 1972 and 1998, the Ministry of Health issued several decrees regulating the number of PAs a pharmacy might employ. For example, in 1992, a pharmacy that grossed between 100 and 200 million CFA was allowed one PA; a pharmacy that grossed between 200 and 300 million was allowed two.[27] At that time the currency had not yet been devalued, and the approximate exchange rate was 300 CFA to US$1. In 1993 the National Order of Pharmacists recorded the numbers of PAs employed by certain pharmacies as follows: Pharmacie Kermel (2), Pharmacie Point E (1), Pharmacie Nouvelle (1), Pharmacie Bel-Air (2), Pharmacie Guigon (2), Pharmacie Drugstore (2).[28]

The subsequent devaluation of the CFA severely affected the Senegalese economy and led to changes in pharmacy regulation and management. By 1998, with the devaluation and subsequent weakening of the local currency coupled with the strength of the United States dollar, the approximate exchange rate was 550 CFA to US$1. The threshold at which a pharmacy was allowed to hire a PA had also increased, to a gross income of 272.2 million CFA. Those that were able to do so had maintained their vitality despite changes in legislation and economic challenges. These figures indicate the economic security of Senegal's pharmacy owners, which is significant in a country where in the mid-1990s, per capita GDP was $1200, or 600,000 CFA, and 50 percent of the population lived in poverty. It is even more significant in a country where despite poverty, low levels of literacy, and women's social limitations, women are able to own the majority of pharmacies in the greater Dakar metropolitan area.

Globalization and Senegal's Pharmacy Sector: Pharmaceutical Distribution and Importation

Pharmacy owners also had to respond to the many (and interrelated) national and international policies influencing pharmacy practice and the pharmaceutical sector. Senegal's public health sector consists of state-managed hospitals, pharmaceutical depots, and clinics in addition to private pharmacies, medical offices, and clinics. The national government devotes about 5 percent of its budget to the health care system. Senegal also receives a significant amount of foreign aid from the French government, USAID, and a number of nongovernmental organizations (NGOs), such as Africare, Oxfam, the World Bank, and the United Nations Development Programme. By the 1990s, approximately one-half of the funds allotted to promoting public health were being distributed to the private health care sector. The National Pharmaceutical Suppliers (Pharmacie national d'approvisionnement, PNA) acquires drugs from foreign and local manufacturers and distributes them to the public and para-public sectors of the Senegalese system. Since the inception of the 1987 Bamako Initiative, which aimed to decentralize and improve access to health care in West Africa, it has supplied low-cost generic drugs to public facilities. It has been quite controversial, however, as it often runs low on stock and its distribution networks are unreliable.

In 1969, Marc Sankalé found that that the majority of drugs on the African continent were still imported from Europe. Senegalese figures from 1970 support this claim and show that, a decade after decolonization, 98 percent of all drugs in Senegal were imported from France. In 1981, 95 percent were still imported, with 90 percent originating in France. Not much had changed by 2000, when 85 percent of the drugs in Senegal came from France and 5 percent from other countries; only 10 percent originated in Senegal.[29] The majority of the locally produced drugs had been in use for decades and were among the least expensive; many pharmacists sold them at little or no markup, forgoing profit for public health.

Three corporations, Laborex, COPHASE, and Sodipharm, coordinate the distribution of drugs to private pharmacies in Senegal. Laborex controls about 60 percent of the market and grossed more than US$40 million in 2000. Approximately 85 percent of the drugs used in the public sector, and 90 percent of those in the private sector, are imported from abroad, usually from France. Additionally, a few companies manufacture drugs in Senegal, such as Industrial Pharmaceutical Suppliers of West Africa (Société industrielle pharmaceutique de l'Ouest africain, SIPOA) (which is Senegalese-owned), Parke Davis, and Sanofi-Aventis.

Some respondents who participated in this project were frustrated by their dependence on foreign pharmaceuticals and called for more to be produced locally. They often cited Morocco and Algeria as examples of countries with greater autonomy in this area. From the mid-1960s to the mid-1980s, Morocco expanded and diversified its production of pharmaceuticals. The project was so successful that Morocco is classified as a European drug supplier, and the country now supplies drugs to North Africa, sub-Saharan Africa, and Western Europe. N'deye Toutane Ngom passionately decried Senegal's dependence on French drugs, asking, "If the French impose an embargo on Senegal—what we will do in terms of pharmaceuticals?"[30] Other pharmacists also commented on Senegal's reliance on foreign biomedical production. Khady Bengeloum Diallo argued that the proliferation of French medicines is due to confidence in the quality of French production and that there are pitfalls in diversifying sources: "Counterfeit medicine is a major industry in countries like India. By buying pharmaceuticals from countries that we do not know well, we expose ourselves to increased risks of acquiring counterfeit drugs that may not meet required standards. For this reason, we continue to turn to French laboratories for our supplies."[31] Indeed, counterfeit drugs are manufactured in several of Senegal's new pharmaceutical trade partners, including India, China, and Nigeria; counterfeit production is on the rise in West Africa.[32] Annette Seck N'diaye lamented, "We have the capability here in Senegal. Each year about a hundred pharmacists are trained, and dozens of doctors. Where will they go? About 150–200 pharmacists are currently unemployed. 'C'est le gaspillage' [It is wasteful]. They spend six or seven years studying and then they cannot find employment. We must develop the pharmaceutical industry here in Senegal." She also compared the situation in Senegal with that in Benin. Benin is a smaller country with a smaller number of pharmacists and inhabitants, but it has been able to manufacture one hundred different types of generic drugs.[33]

Scholars have also criticized the dependence of developing countries on Western drug suppliers. Meredith Turshen, for example, discussed many of the difficulties facing developing countries. In particular, she argued that "the 1994 GATT agreements . . . enable large pharmaceutical producers . . . to block third world manufacture of inexpensive pharmaceutical products." In 1999, Turshen found that the United Kingdom, the United States, Germany, Switzerland, and France controlled 75 percent of worldwide pharmaceutical production.[34]

Drug consumption, as well as production, is concentrated in highly developed economies. By the late twentieth century, North America, Europe, and Japan were the largest consumers of pharmaceuticals in the world. In 2003, annual drug sales in the United States totaled $229.5 billion, and in the European Union $115.4 billion. As a result of legislative reforms, the EU has reduced the costs of many of its drugs. As a result, the value of U.S. drug sales, and of profits on them, increased. The United States now "accounts for 46 percent of [worldwide] pharmaceutical sales and 60 percent of the profit."[35]

The dominance of the United States in pharmaceutical production, sales, and policy extends to West Africa. Senegalese producers, for example, are influenced by U.S. commercial pharmaceutical policies, and more U.S. drug companies are lobbying to enter the Senegalese market. Pfizer has already done so. Without massive changes in the local and global pharmaceutical regulating bodies, it is difficult to imagine how Senegal will reduce its reliance on foreign-produced medicine. However, Senegal's primary partner in this trade has been, not the United States, but its former colonizer—France. In her article "Marché des dupes," Diana Senghor heavily criticized Senegal's dependence on French suppliers of medical goods: "Why does Africa continue to receive medicine whose effectiveness is questioned by France's medical corps? In 1979, 1,409 drugs were erased from the list of reimbursable drugs by the health insurers. . . . Thus, a cough syrup (Teyssèdre) is not reimbursable in France, *WHY?* but it is one of the most frequently purchased products in Senegal (it is the third-ranking waste depository for the foreign pharmaceutical industry)."[36] Senghor's findings further demonstrate the dependence of African economies on pharmaceutical imports. This dependency is a legacy of colonialism, and it continues into the twenty-first century.

Pharmacy Regulation and Expansion in Senegal

In addition to facing the challenges created by Senegal's dependence on foreign pharmaceutical manufacturers, pharmacy owners must also confront those posed by the rapidly growing number of people hoping to open new pharmacies of their own. Legislative restrictions on the number, and later the location, of pharmacies continued from the colonial into the postcolonial period. As the population grew and became more concentrated in urban areas, legislation also changed. In the 1970s, one pharmacy was supposed to be constructed for every 15,000 people in greater Dakar.[37] In other regions, there was to be one pharmacy for every 30,000 inhabitants. In fact, in 1979 there was "one pharmacy for every 19,000 inhabitants" between Dakar and Thiès, and countrywide, the figure was "one pharmacy for every 182,000 inhabitants."[38] There were seventy-five pharmacies in all of Senegal, and forty-seven of these were in greater Dakar. More were clearly needed in the less-developed parts of the country outside the urban centers.

In the 1980s, the focus of regulation shifted from population density to the locations of pharmacies and the distance between them. In 1981, the Ministry of Health declared that in greater Dakar (the Cape Verde peninsula) there should be one pharmacy for every 15,000 people, and one for every 30,000 people elsewhere in the country. "The objective is to progressively reduce the ratio to one office for every 10,000 in all the other regions by the year 2000." Additionally, it required pharmacies in downtown Dakar to be at least 1,000 meters apart. Those in metropolitan Dakar were to be at least 1,500 meters apart, and those outside Dakar at least 2,000 meters. Most importantly, it declared that no new pharmacies could be established in downtown Dakar from March 1981 through July 1985.[39] In 1987, in response to the proliferation of pharmacies in the capital, the minister of health recommended to the National Order of Pharmacists that more pharmacies be created outside of greater Dakar.[40] Their distribution improved somewhat in the rural and peri-urban areas, but pharmacies continued to proliferate in Dakar throughout the twentieth century. Many Dakar neighborhoods and suburbs have seen an increase in the number of residents who are professionals or expatriates, with relatively more disposable income. Pharmacists hoping to open pharmacies, who had previously preferred downtown locations, were now drawn to these neighborhoods and suburbs, and their success there led to the foundation of still more.

Pharmaceutical associations closely monitored the distance between pharmacies and the increase in competition as new ones
opened. Sometimes the interests of the state and the pharmacists in-
tersected, but at other times they were at odds with one another. The
minutes of a meeting of members of the National Order of Pharmacists and the Senegalese president, Abdou Diouf, on 21 August 1981
show the two groups cooperating. In addition to agreeing with the
government about the distance between official pharmaceutical distributors, the pharmacists gave examples of pharmacy depots that
had been improperly opened. For example, one had opened in Thiaroye near Pharmacie Thiaroye-sur-Mer. The association claimed that
the pharmacy depot had not followed proper procedure and called
for the state to seek an "immediate solution."[41] Moreover, despite the
law, the proliferation of new pharmacies was not always regulated.
On 1 April 1988, 25 July 1989, and 30 June 1990, the National Order
of Pharmacists sent memos to the Ministry of Health protesting this
rapid expansion. Established pharmacy owners and administrators
were concerned that some new pharmacies were being illegally in-
stalled and the administrators' failure to enforce the law caused difficulties for existing pharmacy owners.[42]

In 1993, at the urging of the National Order of Pharmacists, the
legislation was revised, and in greater Dakar the minimum distance
required between pharmacies was reduced from 1,000 to 350 meters. In the rest of the country, it became 700 meters.[43] This decrease
in spacing had a major impact on the proliferation of pharmacies.
This intervention by the National Order of Pharmacists shows that it
was a powerful lobby for the private pharmaceutical sector. It further
shows how the private sector can leverage its strength against the
public sector, even affecting policies of the Senegalese state.

The number of private pharmacies was also regulated during both
the colonial and the postcolonial period. In 1955, all of Senegal was
allowed a maximum of twenty-nine pharmacies.[44] During the postcolonial period, pharmacies multiplied faster than in the colonial period. In 1979, seventy-five pharmacies existed in Senegal. There were
eighty-two by 1982, and 240 by 2000. Annette Seck N'diaye said that
between 1972 and 2000, the number of pharmacies in Dakar had

grown from thirty to more than 240. These figures were confirmed by calculations that Abdoulahat Mangane and I performed in 2001. Moreover, in 2000, there were a total of 517 pharmacies in Senegal.[45]

In May 2000, 240 of Senegal's 517 pharmacies were situated in greater Dakar. They were everywhere, from the more peripheral neighborhoods of Usine Ben Tally and Scat Urbam to the upper middle-class Point E and the working-class Grand Dakar. Doctors, however, are more concentrated. They are primarily located downtown and in long-established neighborhoods with high median incomes. Pharmacies' greater presence in different regions and neighborhoods helped clients reach them more easily.

While this rapid multiplication of pharmacies increased opportunities for pharmacists during the 1960s, 1970s, and 1980s, by the 1990s many government officials and pharmacists argued that the growth was no longer sustainable. In a letter to the National Order of Pharmacists on 30 June 1990, Minister of Health Marie Mbodji Sarr offered advice to the pharmacy professionals: "The other issue that concerns me is the number of new pharmacies being created. We want to encourage the correct placement of pharmacies to properly supply the population while maintaining cost effectiveness without creating difficulties between existing pharmacies and new pharmacies."[46]

As mentioned, those wishing to open a new pharmacy must receive approval from the National Order of Pharmacists. The officers of the organization approve not only the creation but also the location of the pharmacy. In 1988, fifteen new pharmacies opened in Dakar, and seventy-three in Senegal. In 1990, the order approved nine new pharmacies in Dakar. While these numbers may sound insignificant, Dakar is fairly compact. Neighborhoods like Point E already had several pharmacies; the creation of one or two more often meant trouble for the existing pharmacists. Now they had to compete for customers and profits.

One pharmacist that I interviewed on the outskirts of Point E experienced major financial difficulties because of the reduction of distance between pharmacies. She was not sure if she would be able to stay in business. Conversely, some pharmacists were unable to gain permission to open a pharmacy. Tharcisse Nkulikiyinfura, for instance, made several appeals to open a pharmacy in or near the Sacre-Coeur III neighborhood, to no avail. After he protested that three other pharmacies had opened in the neighborhood, he was finally granted permission.[47] Many of the new pharmacy owners have a relationship with influential pharmacies or high-ranking government officials. By the 1990s, pharmacy ownership could be achieved not only through qualifications but also through nepotism.

Many of the pharmacists interviewed for this project identified the proliferation of pharmacies, the illegal pharmaceutical trade, and the devaluation of the CFA as the greatest challenges of pharmacy ownership. Mariane Coly, owner of Pharmacie du Théâtre and one of the older pharmacists, argued that the market was "almost saturated." Aïssatou Moreau, owner of Pharmacie Chifaoun, elaborated further: "Yes, there are many pharmacies now, and the buying power of consumers has decreased. People are becoming poorer and poorer." Others, like Hawoly Wane Sy, spoke of the changes they had seen: "The profit margins have changed. . . . It is not like my father's generation." Hélène Akindes was one of the most outspoken on this issue, saying that "expansion was the death of pharmacy." As these comments show, pharmacists of all generations felt the effects of the proliferation of pharmacies. Many argued that if the government did not properly regulate their numbers, the profession would decline.[48]

In 2001, Mame Awa Diop, owner of Pharmacie Lat Dior, stated that ten new pharmacies had opened near hers in the last eight years. She argued that pharmacists must operate their pharmacies well to maintain market advantage.[49] As new pharmacies opened, they had to share the customer base with the existing ones. Consumers' buying power did not rise as pharmacies spread, so profits were diluted. Marie Laure Konate, owner of Pharmacie Patte d'oie, argued that early pharmacy owners "worked well" because their pharmacies were well placed, but now, as costs rose and profits shrank, they were increasingly suffering.[50] Khady Bengeloum Diallo also addressed these issues. She said, "It is necessary that the state regulate the expansion of pharmacies. One finds pharmacies on every street corner, and this is apparently making the profession more difficult. Pharmacy graduates are also having more difficulty [in finding work] after they complete their studies."[51]

In contrast, a few pharmacy owners said that these changes in legislation and the growth of pharmacy ownership were beneficial. Oumy Ndoye Fall, owner of Pharmacie Diraaf Mboye Ndoye, told her story: "Recent changes allowed for the creation of many more pharmacies. I applied to open a pharmacy in 1989 when I graduated but I had to wait seven years . . . eight years for another chance to open a pharmacy. They changed the legislation and liberalized it, thereby helping my authorization."[52] From the 1920s until the 1950s, pharmacy enrollments and graduation rates were low. These numbers began to increase in the 1960s, but in the 1970s and 1980s, they grew at an unprecedented pace. For example, between 1950 and 1952, only eight pharmacists completed their studies. In 1961, forty-eight pharmacy students graduated; in 1971, there were 214; in 1981, 701; and in 1991, fully 1,110.[53] The liberalization of public health policy and education reforms in the first decades of the postcolonial government helped to encourage students to complete college and graduate studies. In addition, as the numbers of pharmacies grew, many observers were drawn by the possibility of a lucrative career.

Despite the many difficulties of pharmacy ownership, many of the pharmacists succeeded in business and maintained professional goodwill. Informants were asked what strategies they employed to achieve this. Most said that in order to be successful they had to successfully manage their staff, maintain honest relationships with customers, and keep regular hours at their pharmacies. Rokhaya Guéye, owner of Pharmacie Cheikh Ibrahima Diallo, said that "good marketing, presence in the pharmacy, good relationships with clients, and good professional character" were keys to success. Bineta Dia, owner of Pharmacie Coope, agreed that "good counsel to clients" and a female pharmacist helped to sustain success. Marie Laure Konate, owner of Pharmacie Patte d'oie, added that pharmacists must pay their suppliers and employees on time.[54]

Other pharmacists spoke highly of their choice of profession: "It is a good profession. My relationship with the public is very good and I offer lots of counsel." Mariane Coly said that her "contact with clientele" offered the most satisfaction. Khady Bengeloum Diallo also spoke of the gratification that she received in interacting with her customers. She believed that customers gravitated to pharmacies because they found pharmacists more accessible than hospital officials. "For this reason the population holds greater affinity for and confidence in us."[55]

Pharmacy clients include people from different ethnic groups and both genders. Middle-class and affluent clients tend to visit pharmacies more regularly because of their greater resources. In addition, many of those in higher socioeconomic strata use their ability to buy pharmaceuticals to reinforce their status. They are less likely to delay buying medicines for minor illness, and more likely to buy multiple versions of a drug and luxury items such as diet pills. In addition, the affluent of Senegal, like their counterparts throughout sub-Saharan Africa, have become more prone to "diseases of affluence" like diabetes and hypertension, making them more likely to pursue sustained biomedical interventions.

As shown, many pharmacists found job satisfaction in counseling and interacting with their clientele. Many of them spoke about being proud of contributing to public health and offering affordable health care options. At the same time, the coexistence of traditional healing practices was also important. While most pharmacists did not officially support cooperation between biomedical and complementary approaches, they were aware that clients often visited traditional healers before or at the same time as seeing them. In Senegal, *pharmacopée* (herbal healing) is usually attributed to practitioners and remedies found outside the pharmacy, though a few pharmacies (largely those catering to expatriate communities, like Pharmacie Guigon) stock a variety of herbal remedies. The majority of these remedies are imported from Western countries.

Like other health care providers, pharmacists are aware that their clients pursue multiple strategies, and factor this into their interactions with them. When I asked my informants about the impact of *pharmacopée* on biomedical pharmacy, most said that plant-based remedies were popular and that clients routinely preferred them to biomedical pills, tinctures, and similar offerings. Some pharmacists even sold herbal medicines, and others argued for more engagement between biomedical and traditional health practitioners. Many of my respondents were concerned that Senegal had no formal system for certifying herbal drugs and healers, and thus supported a policy of marketing proven herbal remedies and creating a network of reputable traditional health practitioners. Pharmacists respond to economic devaluations, consumers' concurrent use of herbal medicine, and other local and global developments in a variety of innovative ways.

5 Pharmaceutical Trafficking in Colonial and Postcolonial Senegal

But in Africa, the interaction between the practice of power, war, economic accumulation, and illicit activities of various types forms a particular political trajectory which can be fully appreciated only if it is addressed in historical depth.

—Jean-François Bayart, Stephen Ellis, and Beatrice Hibou

Four years after Senegal was granted independence, an American scholar, Harold Wilensky, wrote a provocative essay on the process of achieving professional status in the United States. Wilensky discussed how political and organizational barriers inhibited some American occupations from achieving professional status. He concluded, "If the marks of a profession are a successful claim to exclusive technical competence and adherence to the service ideal, the idea that all occupations move toward professional authority— this notion of the professionalization of everyone—is a bit of sociological romance."[1] Just as it did for some fields in the United States, the professionalization of pharmacy in Senegal would take time and perseverance.

Most significantly for pharmacists, the new government of Senegal failed to firmly and clearly regulate who could and could not represent themselves as health care professionals. Street pill peddlers, black-market drug traffickers, counterfeit or fake drugs, and a two-tier drug market (formal and informal) challenged pharmacists' authority. It took time before Senegalese pharmacists could protect and defend their domain. Pharmacists, however, were not romantic but pragmatic about the challenges they faced in postcolonial Senegal. Over the *longue durée* of Francophone West African pharmacy practice, pharmacists have confronted diverse professional constraints and opportunities.

From the advent of pharmacy training in the French colony, there were constraints on education and funding. By the end of the twentieth century, however, two of the more prominent challenges to pharmacy ownership were the proliferation of pharmacies that resulted from the loosening of zoning and licensing laws, and the illegal trade in pharmaceuticals. The latter has existed for many decades in different forms. Because pharmaceutical trafficking profoundly complicates business management and local and global health security, this chapter begins to reconstruct the illegal pharmaceutical trade from the early decades of the twentieth century through an examination of colonial documents, oral interviews, and other primary materials.

Informal Trade Markets in Sahelian and Sub-Saharan Africa

Pharmaceutical trafficking, or the illegal trade in drugs, consists of the acquisition, transportation, or distribution of controlled drugs without the required license or government authorization. The drugs themselves are legal to consume, although their distribution can be legal or illegal depending on how it is done. Francophone West Africa has a long history of illegal pharmaceutical trade. As early as the 1940s, colonial officials were documenting it throughout West Africa. In the early decades of the trade, those implicated were primarily French colonial medical officials and independent traders. By the 1980s, Africans, particularly Senegalese, Nigerians, and Gambians, who were all involved in transregional networks, dominated the trade in Senegal. In reconstructing these changes over time, I show the transformation of the trade's investors as well as the expansion of its global connections.

My work builds on recent studies that have addressed the illegal flow of women, children, and weapons, as well as illicit drugs. In "Spaces of Engagement: How Borderlands, Illegal Flows, and Territorial States Interlock," Willem van Schendel discusses the difficulty of assessing these networks of illegal trade, arguing that borderlands "provide an excellent site to study the intermingling and overlapping of various legal and illegal flows," and that others may perceive these illegal activities as legitimate.[2] Many of Africa's illegal transnational networks rely on the instability of borderlands, poor government enforcement, political corruption, informal markets, and social transition to thrive. Most drugs in Senegal's parallel market are transferred from borderlands or other unregulated territories to urban sites. Drugs enter Senegal via ancient trans-Saharan routes or newer trading networks, and by automobile, boat, and plane. Once they enter the country, their subsequent transfers are less regulated.

In the past two decades, research interest in the illicit trade in drugs has grown. Several recent theses have tackled this topic in Côte d'Ivoire, Cameroon, Niger, and Senegal. They analyze the influence of this trade on public health and society through the lens of biomedical study and show how public health security in these countries is affected by the sale of illegally trafficked pharmaceuticals.[3]

The routes of the illegal trade in pharmaceuticals overlap with those of the illegal trade in other goods and in people: undocumented migrants, and women and children who are trafficked as domestics or sex slaves. In *The Criminalization of the State in Africa*, Jean François Bayart, Stephen Ellis, and Beatrice Hibou address kleptocracy, the criminalization of goods, and informal transnational trade, and argue that it is difficult to create a quantifying mechanism to identify criminality in Africa.[4] The formal and the informal intersect in certain pharmaceutical transactions. This chapter extends Jean and John Comaroff's ideas about the intersections of the legal, extralegal, and criminal and it also examines shifts in what "illegal" means in colonial French West Africa and independent Senegal.[5] A 2004 issue of *Politique africaine* addressed a number of extralegal economic activities, including counterfeiting and the trade in psychotropic drugs.[6] A few studies have examined pharmaceutical trafficking in specific parts of the continent and as a part of larger investigations.[7] Others have probed the trade in psychotropic drugs in West Africa and the Maghreb.[8]

All of these works document the existence of illegal trading networks in Africa and inform my analysis of pharmaceutical trading networks in this chapter. I examine shifts in what "illegal" means in colonial French West Africa and independent Senegal. In particular, I ask who determines the criminality of the sale of pharmaceuticals. This chapter examines the historical trajectory of drug trafficking through the lens of illegal pharmaceutical distribution in French West Africa and postcolonial Senegal. It deepens our understanding of what materials have been trafficked as drugs in African history.

Despite the rich historical literature on colonial medicine, public health, and pharmacopoeia, few scholars have published on Senegal's involvement in the illegal trade in pharmaceutical drugs.[9] Didier Fassin, the first scholar to examine the illegal pharmaceutical trade, published on the topic in the 1980s and 1990s. He identified the trade in contraband pharmaceuticals in the course of a larger study of the Senegalese public health sector. His work also considered many of the larger, even global, implications of the trade.[10] However, most of the trafficked goods and people intersect and mingle along global trade routes.[11] In a 2010 article, I revisited Fassin's findings and expanded upon them to consider not only regional but transregional networks in Europe and Asia. I also analyzed another manifestation of this illegal trade in the form of Keur Serigne Bi, an illegal market devoted primarily to the resale of stolen pharmaceuticals.[12]

Similarly, although studies have been published of the sale of narcotics and other psychotropic drugs in other parts of sub-Saharan Africa, especially Anglophone countries in East and West Africa, only a few scholars have addressed the issue in Senegal.[13] Jean-François Werner is one of them. In *Marges, sexe, et drogues à Dakar,* he investigates the trade in illicit street drugs, along with prostitution and other illegal activities, in Pikine, a suburb of Dakar. It is important that scholars begin examining these issues in the Senegambian subregion, but they must also consider the comparative historiographies and global intersections of the narcotics trade. Sales of illicit drugs and extralegal pharmaceuticals are inextricably linked to global developments.

While most of the discussion of the illegal pharmaceutical trade looks at recent decades, my research shows that the illegal trade in pharmaceuticals began in French West Africa in the 1940s, which is when the earliest records of it appear. Like the locally established trade in illicit psychotropic drugs, it was of major concern to French colonial officials. It involved the illegal acquisition and sale of goods, and also questions about who was and was not authorized to sell pharmaceuticals. Most correspondence and legislation regarding regulation of this trade originated in Dakar, as it was the capital of French West Africa. Most of the pharmacy inspectors and other high-ranking medical personnel were also based in Senegal. In the early decades, the illegal pharmaceutical trade was controlled by French nationals and French expatriates living in the colony. Some pharmacists also participated in the illegal trade to increase their profits.

On 23 August 1950, Dr. Garcin, the director general of public health, sent a letter to the high commissioner of French West Africa regarding pharmaceutical trafficking in Côte d'Ivoire. He said that it was difficult for him to enforce the 1926 laws regulating pharmacies in French West Africa. Pharmacists were increasingly evading the restrictions on controlled drugs by buying them from authorized importers and reselling them themselves illegally. Despite periodic visits by pharmacy inspectors and calls for greater vigilance, the resale of such pharmaceuticals persisted. Because of this, Dr. Garcin called for the importation of drugs to be better documented and records kept of their circulation.[14] In Abidjan, Côte d'Ivoire, in 1950, the head of pharmacy, Mr. Perrotto, asked public health officials to pay special attention to the resale of pharmaceuticals, reminding them that these resales were illegal.[15] Pharmacies also sometimes sold drugs to each other, avoiding the official distribution networks.

French colonial officials did try to reduce the illegal trade in pharmaceuticals. In a letter to an administrator in Dakar, Dr. Garcin offered a number of suggestions. They included more vigilantly monitoring imported "toxic medicine" and "narcotics" and further restricting the right to import these drugs. He proposed that certain prescriptions be required to originate in France and that importers be required to show customs officials their import permit from the pharmacy inspector; otherwise the package would be sent back.[16] In the most egregious cases, sanctions would be laid against offending pharmacists, limiting their professional activity.

On 12 August 1950, the governor of Côte d'Ivoire sent a letter to the governor general of French West Africa in which he said that Pharmacie du Serpent in Lyon, France, had sent twenty-five tubes of Dagenan and a shipment of Stovarsol to Morifere Soumahero, a businessman in Gagnoa, Côte d'Ivoire.[17] Both drugs were considered highly toxic and had been identified as dangerous as early as 1926. Dagenan is a sulfonamide antibiotic; it can cause serious side effects and interact dangerously with other drugs. Derived from arsenic, Stovarsol is used to treat various stages of syphilis, lupus, and several parasitic infections. It was developed in 1921 at one of the Pasteur Institutes. These two powerful drugs have historically been strongly regulated because of their potency and the severity of their side effects. In fact, in some countries their use is discouraged and less potent alternatives are recommended. Misuse can lead to the development of antibiotic-resistant bacteria, but also, especially with Stovarsol, to physical impairment and death.

In October 1950, the governor general wrote again, this time to the high commissioner of France. He noted that although the shipment of these drugs from France to Côte d'Ivoire appeared illegal, neither customs agents nor inspectors had the legal power to prevent the importation of drugs that were not on the list of approved drugs. For this reason, he requested the right to authorize them to seize "dangerous" and "toxic" medicines, such as were being distributed in this case.[18]

Other cases found in the archives are much more complicated and include multiple forms of illegal trading. A 1951 memo from one pharmacy inspector to another on the traffic in pharmaceutical products illustrates the variety of possibilities. Georges Kintogbe, a merchant based in the city of Cotonou in Dahomey (Benin), was implicated in illegal sales of not only pharmaceuticals but also Citroën trucks. Without a license, he was trading in Stovarsol, Dagenan, mercury, and other highly regulated and controlled medicines, and also in pharmaceutical supplies, including syringes and needles. When discovered, he had been selling drugs for more than six years in French and British colonies: Togo, Dahomey, and Nigeria.[19]

Kintogbe's activities in the illegal medicine trade did not exist in a vacuum. His network was vast, with many suppliers and accomplices in both the colonies and the metropole. As inspectors realized the scale of the trade, they discovered that drugs were being transported both by land and by air, on Air France, Aéro Africaine, and other airlines. In France, several pharmacists were supplying medicine for Georges Kintogbe's business, including M. H. Garraud in Bordeaux and F. Taulelle in Lyon. Taulelle was infamous; he had been implicated in multiple cases of illegal pharmaceutical trading. This multinational trafficking was apparently quite successful; the authorities were able to intercept almost eight hundred packages of pharmaceuticals in Cotonou and Ouidah.[20] Given the many streams of Kintogbe's business and the length of time he had been engaged in it, it is clear that this case represents only a small fraction of the trade.

Morifere Soumahero and Georges Kintogbe were two of a few African merchants who were cited in illegal pharmaceutical distribution. As the records show, they were able to engage in this traffic through business alliances with French pharmacists and other medical personnel. Many of these alliances were transnational, with drugs being transferred directly from the metropole to the colony for illegal distribution. Several pharmacies and laboratories in Bordeaux, Lyon, Paris, and Marseille were implicated in the trade.

These examples show that the categories of legal and illegal were not fixed, and colonial officials and inspectors had a range of options in enforcing the law. They raise questions about what categories of drugs could be sold legally, in a pharmacy, and about who had the authority to sell and resell them. It is also evident that the regulations lacked power and were difficult for colonial officials to enforce. French and African pharmacists and pharmacy assistants continued to skirt the law in efforts to maximize profits and meet demand.

Pharmaceutical Trafficking in the Colony and the Postcolony

During the colonial era, the pharmaceutical trade was virtually controlled by French pharmaceutical companies and colonial bureaucrats. Illegal pharmaceutical trafficking could mean trading outside of official state-sanctioned networks, selling psychotropic drugs, or selling drugs without being licensed to do so. While some of the recipients of the illegally trafficked drugs were African, most of the players were French nationals. The colonial machine controlled not only political decisions in the colony but also the dissemination of biomedical care and knowledge. Most of the extant correspondence originated with colonial officials in the colony or the metropole; only a few sources include the voices of pharmacists responding to state regulation. Moreover, the archive is largely silent on the trade in pharmaceuticals in the colonial and postcolonial periods, although more documentation exists on that in psychoactive drugs. By using oral interviews, organizational reports, and site visits, this chapter provides a greater diversity of voices, particularly those of Africans.

In the 1950 and 1960s, as Africans became more prominent in the profession of pharmacy, they began to take greater interest in legal and extralegal pharmaceutical trades. Nonetheless, even after independence in 1960 French expatriates continued to dominate the pharmaceutical industry. As explained later in this chapter, during this period the Mouride brotherhood, an Islamic Sufi order, was at the pinnacle of its economic power. The brotherhood's economic power, its efforts to diversify its investments, and the shifting postcolonial climate all created opportunities for others to enter the pharmaceutical market. As a result, Africans came to dominate the parallel pharmaceutical trade. Further, the illegal trafficking of pharmaceuticals came to include their acquisition by illegal means, shipment on illegal networks, and sale in illegal markets.

In postcolonial Senegal, new questions arose: who controls pharmaceutical networks? Does the origin of a drug determine its legitimacy? What is the proper role of government in the regulation of drugs? How do pharmacists compete with informal parallel markets, which may be fixed or transient? How do they compete with a politically powerful religious organization, the Mouride brotherhood, which is partially protected by the state?

The political and economic transformations in the decades surrounding independence extended to the pharmaceutical sector. As described in earlier chapters of this book, the number of Senegalese pharmacists and pharmacy owners increased rapidly in the 1960s, 1970s, and 1980s. The numbers of French expatriates were decreasing, and most professions were becoming Africanized. French nationals and their contacts in the metropole lost control not only of local formal enterprises but also of many extralegal activities, including the illegal trafficking of pharmaceuticals. In 1976, the Senegalese state made pharmaceuticals tax-exempt, which led to a significant increase in their importation from France and other countries. At the same time, pharmaceutical trafficking became more profitable. As a result, it was entrenched in Senegal by the late 1980s. This rise in the parallel sale of pharmaceuticals coincided with increases in literacy, the diversification of certain formal and informal sectors, and greater trust in biomedical treatment. Thus, a new market of consumers arose, which benefited both formal sectors of the pharmaceutical industry and those who sold drugs illegally. In particular, the Mouride brotherhood was extending and diversifying its commercial interests in the country and the region, and pharmaceutical trafficking became a large part of its portfolio.

Mouride Power and Economic Diversification

Cheikh Anta Bamba Mbacké, or Amadou Bamba, founded the Mouride Sufi order in the 1880s. Loosely structured at its origins, it rapidly gained adherents and gradually became a highly organized brotherhood, which appealed to a wide segment of Senegalese society. French bureaucrats began consolidating and extending their subregional colonial policy in the late nineteenth century, and they encountered opposition from a number of religious and political leaders, including Lat Dior (d. 1886) and El Hajj Umar Tall (d. 1864). Such encounters with Muslim leaders would influence France's policy toward the Mouride brotherhood.

As a direct result of France's expansionist policies, Cheikh Amadou Bamba was removed from the immediate region. He was exiled to Gabon from 1895 to 1902 and to Mauritania from 1903 to 1907. Touba, Senegal, the Mouride brotherhood's capital city, and "Islam became a unifying force for a defeated people."[21] The Mourides were a potential religious threat to the French, as some of their doctrines fomented cultural and social conflict. Cheikh Babou explains that the brotherhood "championed values and behavior that antagonized the French civilizing mission. Drawing from Amadou Bamba's Sufi doctrine and Wolof cultural values, it put community above the individual, it valued wealth sharing over accumulation, it promoted loyalty to religious guides, discouraged rebellion against colonial rulers, [but] encouraged withdrawal and distance from anything related to the administration." Although the Wolof sometimes used French cultural markers, they tended toward conservatism. They spoke their own language and promoted the wearing of traditional clothing, and although they may have written letters on letterhead and mailed them with stamps, they used Arabic script.[22] The Mourides were able to straddle different cultures as they saw fit. In colonial and postcolonial Senegal, they applied this syncretic approach to their commercial interests.

In addition to religious activity, the Mourides were highly engaged in agricultural production and the acquisition of capital through mass merchant migration.[23] Initially, they controlled much of Senegalese peanut farming. They also orchestrated most of the parallel cross-border trade in drugs in the West African subregion. This economic power gave them considerable influence with the colonial government. In their raw and processed forms, peanuts and peanut oil were exported throughout Africa and to European markets. As the Mourides gradually extended their control over peanut production, they became more interested in maintaining their economic influence than in initiating conflict with the French. The brotherhood's leaders contented themselves with indirect rule of Touba and its environs.

By World War II, the brotherhood had more than seventy thousand followers, and in 2000, the number topped 3 million.[24] As its numbers grew, many members migrated to far-flung urban centers such as New York, Dubai, Marseille, Tokyo, and Milan in search of new trade opportunities. They used their accumulated capital and knowledge of global markets to invest foreign capital in innovative ways. In addition to pharmaceuticals, the Mourides formally and informally imported and exported a variety of products, including electronics, music, food, and household appliances.

In "Africa's Frontiers in Flux," Achille Mbembe defines Touba as a "warehouse town" and describes the transformations of regional and global networks, saying that "new and unexpected forms of territoriality . . . have appeared, with their boundaries not necessarily matching the official limits, norms or languages of the states."[25] These informal networks are critical to the illegal pharmaceutical trade, since they are analogous to other illicit trade routes. In considering these informal trade activities, Christian Coulon and Donal Cruise O'Brien describe Touba as "a veritable clandestine Harrods, Senegalese style, which the state cannot keep under control without angering the head of the brotherhood."[26] Thus, Touba's protected position coupled with Mouride commercial ingenuity has fueled the brotherhood's investment in Senegal's parallel markets. Touba is a perfect example of an extraterritorial space that does not have to conform to the social and geopolitical boundaries of the Senegalese state.

The Clandestine Trade in Pharmaceuticals

In the last decade of the twentieth century Touba, the second largest city in Senegal, had a population of approximately 1 million, but the city contained only eleven official pharmacies and a partially constructed hospital.[27] In comparison, Dakar, with a population of 2 million, housed more than two hundred pharmacies.[28] Upon examination, it is clear that in Touba, facilities other than pharmacies sell pharmaceuticals. The city contains 250 pharmaceutical depots that are targeted by participants in the larger illegal trade nexus, who siphon off supplies and sell them in other parts of the country. The ubiquity of these depots indicates the informal nature of public health services in Touba. This informal approach to public health is also evident in how members of the Mouride brotherhood invest in and manage pharmaceutical trade networks. For most of its existence, Touba operated outside official state regulation. This lack of regulation allowed its denizens to freely pursue formal and informal business activities with limited risk. Extralegal activities like selling pharmaceutical drugs in informal economies were often considered innovative and entrepreneurial but not criminal. In general, low literacy rates, unfamiliarity with drug safety, and economic uncertainty in Senegal and many other African countries contribute to the flourishing of alternative pharmaceutical networks.

While the parallel trade in pharmaceuticals has existed for many years, the problem in Senegal was exacerbated after the January 1994 devaluation of the currency. It created an economic crisis in Senegal and reduced the buying power of the population. It also extended the reach of the parallel market in three ways. First, straitened consumers assumed that they would save money by buying biomedical drugs from an alternative source. Second, the loans that pharmacy owners had taken to buy property, stock, and other items doubled in cost, which meant they had to increase prices in order to make payments. Finally, third, many of the investors in the parallel market took advantage of these changing conditions.

Drugs involved in this market are obtained in a variety of ways. Medicines originating in countries other than France and Senegal are obtained through transnational networks. Two of the most prominent originate in Gambia and Nigeria. The Mouride brotherhood purchases drugs directly from two state-sponsored wholesalers, National Pharmaceutical Suppliers (PNA) and Industrial Pharmaceutical Suppliers of West Africa (SIPOA), even though they are meant for sale in Senegal's pharmacies, hospitals, and rural dispensaries.[29] Drugs are also obtained by stealing parts of pharmaceutical shipments while they are in the port of Dakar. The Mouride brotherhood and some foreign countries, including Gambia, are directly implicated in these thefts. Because they affect the regional trade in pharmaceuticals, they have led to calls to further secure seaports, as well as land and air trade routes.

Keur Serigne Bi: A Parallel Marketplace

In *Pouvoir et maladie en Afrique,* Didier Fassin describes the three primary types of illegal sellers in this region as "those who sell in established markets . . . [those who sell in] fixed locations such as street corners . . . [and] ambulatory vendors."[30] One of the most important established markets in Senegal is Keur Serigne Bi, a market in central Dakar whose name means "the house of the *serigne,*" or religious leader. It is by far the most notorious place to purchase biomedical pharmaceuticals outside a pharmacy. Its existence delights bargain hunters, informal traders, and investors, while simultaneously frustrating Senegal's public health institutions.

It is not easy to define Keur Serigne Bi. A passer-by happening upon it by accident would probably not afford it much attention. No signs alert the buyer who approaches the wall surrounding this informal pharmaceutical market. A few traders are stationed on the sidewalk outside, and they sell items that would likely be found in a U.S. supermarket's over-the-counter aisle, such as cold remedies and pain medication. The most popular drugs sold on the street in Senegal are painkillers, antibiotics, antimalarial agents, psychotropic "prescription" drugs, and skin bleaching creams.[31] Many of these items are imported from countries such as China and Nigeria that have not historically been associated with Senegal's legal pharmaceutical market. Pills are not always found in their original packaging and may be sold individually. Many of the small-scale traders outside Keur Serigne Bi would not arouse any suspicion, as similar scenes appear throughout western Africa. Tables with minor pharmaceuticals are common in markets and on certain streets. In addition, many neighborhood *boutiques* (convenience stores) will provide basic medicines, so the uninitiated may remain unaware of what hides behind the wall.

An entrance on Blaise Diagne Avenue invites more serious customers into a courtyard that leads to stalls. The layout of Keur Serigne Bi is maze-like. On the surface, it looks like an enormous compound or small trading venue. In fact, it is a pharmaceutical market controlled primarily by investors from the Mouride brotherhood. The traders look rather inconspicuous and are less aggressive than other local hawkers. They may not approach a customer but rather wait to be approached. While many of the sellers are Senegalese and most are Mouride, some come from other West African countries.

On one visit to Keur Serigne Bi, I investigated the pharmaceutical products that were available. A Senegalese colleague and I walked through the market's labyrinth. Most of the stalls and rooms were closed, and the sellers stood outside guarding their merchandise. Because of periodic raids by police and other government officials, the vendors do not want to attract suspicion. We approached one seller, who asked in Wolof to see a prescription. I replied that I did not have one, but would like to see his products. He appeared cautious but allowed us to view his merchandise. Shelves around the walls of the stalls contain hundreds of pharmaceuticals. When a customer comes with a prescription, the seller matches it with a product. However, most of the consumers who visit the market do not bring prescriptions; they choose their own medicine.

Consumers who visit Keur Serigne Bi to treat an illness often justify buying there by saying that prices are lower. In fact, the price difference between drugs sold in the formal sphere and the informal sphere is minimal, and drugs are sometimes slightly more expensive at Keur Serigne Bi than in pharmacies. Because most of the market's customers tend to avoid pharmacies, they are unaware of this. Just as they do not visit pharmacies, in most cases they do not visit doctors. The sellers may also diagnose and suggest treatments, which may be incorrect or inappropriate. Most of the sellers at Keur Serigne Bi are semiliterate and have no pharmaceutical training, and their ignorance can lead them to exacerbate existing illnesses or create new health concerns.

Sellers have different reasons for participating in the parallel pharmaceutical market. Like itinerant and market sellers on the continent and abroad, they hope to improve their economic livelihood. In his book *Money Has No Smell: The Africanization of New York City,* Paul Stoller explores the ethics of informal sales transactions. Stoller found that West African Muslim sellers (some of them members of the Mouride brotherhood) felt that because the products they sold were not illegal, and they used the money to support their families and religious institutions, there was nothing improper in their trading methods.[32] Sellers at Keur Serigne Bi often express similar ideas. They describe the illegally acquired pharmaceuticals that they sell as "licit" and not "illicit." Increasingly, however, African governments, medical professionals, NGOs and other organizations, and international policing communities condemn their activities as criminal. Formal and informal markets appear to disagree about what defines criminality. Perhaps in the Senegalese imaginary, this definition will become more distinct if the government attacks the illegal trade in pharmaceuticals more forcefully. At present, whenever the closing of Keur Serigne Bi is ordered, it always manages to reopen. The government does not confiscate the sellers' stock, and the sellers eventually reestablish their networks and continue to trade in pharmaceuticals.

Other Markets: Keur Serigne Yi

In addition to Keur Serigne Bi, there are three similar markets in Dakar, located in the center of the city and in the suburbs of Pikine and Thiaroye. These markets are major suppliers of diverse goods, including pharmaceuticals and consumer goods. Located near Keur Serigne Bi in Dakar proper, Sandaga is the largest market in town. It is a center for the sale of both local and imported goods and services, including domestic and imported cloth, electronics, cassette tapes, art, ready-made clothes, foodstuffs, and other goods. Some of these items are authentic, and others are contraband or counterfeit. Like

Keur Serigne Bi, Sandaga is controlled by the Mourides. It developed from the migrations of the Mouride traders from Touba to other Senegalese cities. This makes it an obvious venue for the brotherhood's extension of its enterprise to the sale of illegally traded pharmaceuticals. When asked about Keur Serigne Bi in an interview, a respondent replied, "Keur Serigne yi . . . Il y a maintenant beaucoup," which means "now many exist" in French and Wolof. (In Wolof, *bi* is a singular marker, and *yi* is a plural.).[33] This pharmacist's remark indicates the success of the parallel pharmaceutical trade in Senegal. It also suggests the challenges these illegal activities have created for formal medical sectors. Pharmacists are generally not the beneficiaries of these informal economic exchanges today, as they were in the colonial era.

Residents of Pikine and Thiaroye, many of whom commute to work in Dakar, are generally less educated and less affluent than their urban counterparts. These two suburbs are more violent than the city, and prostitution and the sale of psychotropic drugs and contraband goods, especially electronics such as cellular phones, are common. Medicines, often illegally acquired, and psychotropic drugs are found in local market stalls and are available from salesmen walking the streets. Many of these salesmen seem ill informed about the products they sell. They simply sell the items to make a living. Their stock often changes to meet consumer demand. The drugs sold in these illegal exchanges are distributed through the same parallel networks that support fixed markets such as Keur Serigne Bi.

In the early 1990s, two pharmacy students, Cheikh Tidiane Diaw and Fatou Mbengue, studied pharmaceutical trafficking in urban Senegal. Mbengue's study focused on Dakar and included a small number of informants. She interviewed ambulant pharmaceutical sellers and several stall-keepers at Keur Serigne Bi. She also tested medicine that she purchased on the street for efficacy. Cheikh Diaw conducted a similar study, but one much larger in scope. His study focused on informal trades in Dakar, Kaolack, and Diourbel, and he interviewed 207 ambulant sellers, three-quarters of them male. Both Mbengue and Diaw found that the majority of ambulant sellers were illiterate. Diaw discovered that 23 percent had received no formal education, 67 percent had attended Qur'anic school, 4.8 percent had completed primary school, and 0.4 percent had a secondary education. Many of those who had attended only a Qur'anic school were functionally illiterate. Both researchers also found that many of the sellers knew little about the products that they sold. They educated each other and often conferred with more senior sellers about dosages and side effects.[34] These findings support the concerns of local and international pharmacy associations and NGOs about the dangers of street drugs.

Pharmacy Owners' Reactions to Drug Trafficking

Dakar pharmacists question the efficacy and safety of drugs acquired on the streets from people without pharmaceutical degrees. Many pharmacists acknowledge that the groups who control the pharmaceutical black market collaborate with one another. "It is the Baol-Baol who control it," said one, while others refer to them as "Modou-Modou," or more directly as Mourides.[35] A pharmacist in the Touba region stated that pharmacists sell drugs to nonpharmacists, who then distribute them. Another noted that "the Senegalese who live in other countries and who illegally retrieve pharmaceuticals from these societies" contribute to this trade. Many of the younger pharmacists criticized the situation more directly. D., age 28, who comes from a family of medical professionals, stated that "the Mouride brotherhood, certain pharmacists, certain international organizations, and hospitals" are all involved at some level.[36]

Others supported more stringent regulation and enforcement by the Ministry of Health, the Pharmacy Syndicate, and law enforcement. The National Order of Pharmacists, the Pharmacy Syndicate, and certain individual pharmacists have actively sought to punish sellers in this alternative trade. A group of pharmacists hoping to advance a more stringent antitrafficking campaign with the assistance of the government and a few NGOs created a new organization, the Union of Young Senegalese Pharmacists (Association des jeunes pharmaciens sénégalais, AJPS). In a 2001 report, they called for a "rapid intervention to save the population" and proposed the following interventions:

> The points of sale are known with certainty; people have been identified as suppliers to the illegal pharmaceutical market. The Ministry of Health, Directorate of Pharmacy and Drugs, customs officials, and police need to intervene and show these vendors of death that they cannot resist the iron arm of the State, which strongly shows that it is the protector of its citizens. . . . There must be strong and regular surveillance of Keur Serigne Bi, the markets in Thiaroye, Colobane market, and in Touba. The Directorate of Pharmacy and Drugs must further strengthen its personnel and resources by augmenting the number of inspectors. . . . The customs officials at borders, bridges, and the airport must redouble their efforts and provide systematic searches at the Gambian border. The police and military must not allow any pharmaceutical import which is not authorized by the Directorate of Pharmacy and Drugs.[37]

This report indicates the diversity of the entities engaged in Senegal's parallel market of pharmaceuticals. While some groups and nationalities (the Mouride brotherhood and Gambian nationals) are implicated directly, the local connections to the global traffic in illicit biomedical and psychotropic drugs increased dramatically from the mid-1990s. Most of the pharmacy associations, as well as local and international NGOs, call for points of entry to be better secured. Many members of the Union of Young Senegalese Pharmacists bemoan the lack of direct and sustained intervention by the authorities, the state, and pharmacy associations.

Generic drugs are often a much more affordable alternative to many name-brand drugs to treat ailments like malaria, infection, and iron deficiency. For example, in 2001 a course of treatment with generic amoxicillin cost 1,099 CFA (1.68 euros), while non-generic versions cost between 2,034 and 3,696 CFA (3.10 to 5.63 euros).[38] The market for generic medicine in Africa is not as developed as similar markets in Europe and the United States. Few generic drugs are available, because few drugs are manufactured in Africa, drug distribution is controlled by monopolies, and consumers are poorly educated about generic options and do not understand that they are equivalent to familiar brands. Since the inception of the Bamako Initiative in 1987, sales of drugs by hospitals and pharmacy depots have increased, while pharmacy sales have declined. Many pharmacists have increased their sales of generic drugs, but not all could recover their lost clientele.

Pharmacy and Illegal Provider Encroachment

Many of the pharmacy associations and some individual pharmacists use their professional and personal affiliations to lobby the Senegalese government, the Directorate of Pharmacy, and the Ministry of Health to take stronger positions on drug policy. Arguably, pharmacists have been most effective in their negotiations with the Directorate of Pharmacy. The relationships among the Directorate of Pharmacy, the National Order of Pharmacists, and the Pharmacy Syndicate are intricate and long-standing; they help pharmacists who hope to own and operate pharmacies. Historically, lobbying the state has proved more challenging. While representatives of the Ministry of Health and high-ranking government officials, including presidents and prime ministers, engage the pharmacy lobby, they are slow to accede to the lobby's wishes and have been unable to reduce the illegal trade in pharmaceuticals.

Some of the pharmacists interviewed preferred not to elaborate on this subject and commented only indirectly on how the trade affected their profits. Their reticence likely stems from the implications of Mouride involvement. Not only are the Mourides powerful both politically and economically, but they are also a religious organization. Some of the pharmacists are members of the Mouride brotherhood themselves, while others may not want to criticize such a powerful organization. Even the Senegalese state has been guarded in how it approaches the leaders of the brotherhood. In fact, it is likely that the tepidness of the state's response to the illegal pharmaceutical trade is due to the potential political implications of offending the organization. The marabouts are able to rally votes to support or oppose political leaders from the lowest to the highest levels of the government.

Ways to confront this burgeoning parallel trade in drugs include streamlining the sale of pharmaceuticals in public institutions, such as hospitals and other government-subsidized depots. This would help to ensure drug safety while also reducing retail prices, letting the official networks compete directly with street sellers. Some changes began to be implemented in the 1990s, including public health outreach focused on informing the general population about the hazards of buying medicine on the street. One pharmacist, age 43, who comes from a family of medically trained professionals, argued that there is "no price on health," and that the gravity of the situation demands that people be educated to avoid street drugs, just as they are educated about HIV/AIDS prevention.[39] This pharmacist was one of the most forthcoming critics of formal and informal public health issues, citing local pharmacy activism as a solution to many social ills. Collectively, pharmacists bemoan the authorities' failure to maintain surveillance, and they appeal to police and military officials to block unauthorized pharmaceutical imports.

Organized Local and International Response

Eighteen countries, including Benin, Tunisia, Morocco, Chad, Comoros, Madagascar, and Gabon, sent pharmacist delegates to the pan-African International Pharmaceutical Forum in 2001. On the fourth day of the forum, there was a roundtable discussion on the illegal drug trade. Representatives from all the countries except Gabon acknowledged that this problem exists. Representatives from Guinea estimated that 40 to 45 percent of drug sales had shifted to the informal sector; in Mali, it was estimated that 10 to 30 percent of sales, or 10 million to 30 million CFA, were siphoned off by the illegal pharmaceutical trade.[40]

After discussing the causes of the problem, the pharmacists proposed strategies for solving it. Among these were more collaboration with authorities, surprise visits to "illicit markets," surveillance of trade routes and borders, and better consumer education, especially about the hazards of street drugs. Other strategies offered included making it easier for private pharmacies to buy generics and sell them to consumers, ensuring that pharmacists or licensed assistants were continuously available, reforming the Bamako Initiative, increasing support from the Directorate of Pharmacy, and expanding regulatory mechanisms, including creating an international committee to regulate the parallel market.[41]

While many pharmacists argue that the Senegalese government has responded only weakly to the problem, it has intervened in some ways. The government has participated in various campaigns to educate the public about how to safely buy medicines. Unfortunately, many years often lapse between these campaigns, and many are limited in scope. Further, they are often carried out in French through visual media, especially billboards and advertisements. It may be more effective for the government to pursue campaigns through an audio medium such as radio, and perhaps in Wolof or other local languages.

For years, the National Order of Pharmacists has publicly acknowledged the expansion of this illegal trade, and it has organized several campaigns to reduce it. Some of the people involved in this campaign claim that pharmacists and government officials who are affiliated with this trade obstruct their work. In an interview with *Le soleil* Mamadou Ndiadé, a past president of the National Order of Pharmacists, cited the parallel market as a "major problem," arguing that "not only does the parallel market develop more and more . . . there are other illegal sites for the sale of medicine. There are no measures against Keur Serigne Bi. We fight the battle against this affliction [and] the authorities are also challenged."[42]

In Senegal, while the numbers of informal or illegal sales are much lower, the politics involved are much more nuanced than in many neighboring countries. The powerful Mouride brotherhood has a monopoly on the sale of illegally acquired pharmaceuticals. While many of the drugs are not counterfeit, it is becoming clear that some are. Many members of Senegal's health care community seem torn. While they want to maintain public safety and their own profits, they do not want to take on the Mouride religio-political machine. To be sure, others are members of the Mouride brotherhood and find other conflicts of interest.

Senegalese pharmacists and drug distributors, and the Senegalese government, have all identified a growing need for low-cost medicines, and efforts have been made to provide generic drugs to those in need in many African nations, including in Senegal. Many of the most prescribed drugs have generic equivalents. A few generics are produced in Senegal; others are imported from other African countries and from Europe. The largest suppliers are Morocco and France. The Bamako Initiative outlined ways to provide generic drugs to greater numbers of people, distributing them wholesale to pharmacy depots and hospitals. While consumers in certain areas frequent pharmacy depots, many consumers and pharmacists complain that their stock is unreliable. Many who work in the private arm of the pharmaceutical sector have been lobbying for the right to purchase generic drugs in greater quantities, as those in the public sector can.

Pharmacy owners expressed support for the use of generic drugs; almost all called it a "good thing." While some of them did mention the possibility of selling name-brand drugs to increase profit margins, they honored their oath to protect the population's health. To be sure, the purchase of brand-name drugs is a sign of status. Clients with moderate to high purchasing power will choose a brand name rather than a generic drug. They want to demonstrate their ability to purchase directly from the pharmacy instead of in an informal market. Making generic drugs more available will have little effect on their purchases. However, generics may attract clients who would otherwise have purchased medicine illegally or consulted a traditional healer. Greater publicity and consumer-directed educational campaigns will likely increase the sale of generic drugs.

Regional Implications of Pharmaceutical Trafficking

Pharmacists' concerns have been validated by the growing size of this parallel market. In 1999, Senegal's official pharmaceutical sector grossed approximately 58 billion CFA, or US$83 million.

Ninety-one percent of this, or 52.8 billion CFA, was earned by the private sector. It is estimated that Keur Serigne Bi grossed 6 billion CFA, or almost US$10 million, in the same year. Ten years later, it grossed more than US$8.5 million.[43] This parallel trade makes it difficult to reliably provide medicine in stable, secure environments. In an earlier study of the illegal trade in drugs in Senegal, Fassin argued that the sum of all parallel market sales rivaled that of private pharmacy sales.[44] While it is difficult to accurately estimate the size and impact of the parallel market, undoubtedly it has affected various aspects of the official public health sector.

In the late twentieth century, a variety of campaigns in Francophone Africa tried to reduce illegal drug sales and teach consumers not to self-medicate. Campaigns by ENDA-Tiers Monde and other nongovernmental organizations have attempted to jolt the consumer into avoiding street drugs. In the late 1990s, Côte d'Ivoire recorded and televised illegal transactions in the hopes of raising public consciousness about the dangers of these drugs. In Nigeria, the parallel trade has proven more sinister. Most of the drugs traded in the informal sectors are counterfeit, and counterfeits have significantly infiltrated formal biomedical markets. In the 1980s and 1990s, it was estimated that approximately 50 percent of Nigeria's pharmaceuticals were counterfeit.[45] In response to the growing threat of illegal pharmaceutical sales, Dr. Dora Akunyili, ex-director of Nigeria's National Agency for Food and Drug Administration Control, had more than two dozen sellers convicted and has reviewed and banned dozens of Asian suppliers of counterfeit drugs. In addition, her office has led market raids that have succeeded in reducing the trade in illegal drugs by 80 percent.[46] As a result, Dr. Akunyili became one of the most celebrated fighters against counterfeit drugs in West Africa. But while Nigeria is experiencing some success, countries such as Guinea and Benin are battling seemingly entrenched parallel markets. They are hindered by many factors, including inadequate budgets, corrupt officials, and the political dangers of indicting powerful businessmen.

Senegal has long been connected to larger networks of illegal drug trading. As the seat of French West Africa, it was both a site for drug trafficking and an administrative clearinghouse for the creation of policy and the initiation of attempts to control and prevent illegal activity. As the pharmaceutical profession progressed and markets diversified, the legal status of various drugs changed. In the transition from colonialism to postcolonialism, these statuses were further confused. Like many sectors of the formal economy, the informal economy became Africanized, meaning that African merchants and businessmen, and the Mouride brotherhood, made major investments in the parallel pharmaceutical trade. While aware of this transnational pharmaceutical trafficking, the Senegalese government was not able to contain it.

The analysis presented in this chapter is critical to a larger understanding of the intersection of globalization and public health policy in colonial and postcolonial contexts. It shows how pharmacists respond to these challenges through individual initiative and collective action as well as through interactions with clients and the government.

Postscript

In the summer of 2009, Senegal's pharmacists shuttered their pharmacies, took to the streets, and held a rally at the headquarters of the National Order of Pharmacists. These protests were held in response to a robbery and murder at Pharmacie Actuel, one of hundreds of robberies of Senegal's pharmacies since 2006. Pharmacy owners viewed the murder of the owner's nephew as a symptom of the encroachment of the illegal pharmaceutical trade on biomedical pharmacies. It marked the nadir of negotiations between pharmacy associations, the Senegalese state, and illegal traders, and it spurred pharmacists to rally to regain control of their livelihoods. In 2010, the physical structure housing Keur Serigne Bi was destroyed by arson. Investors in the institution continue to regroup, and trade has resumed in nearby buildings and surrounding streets. The parallel trade in pharmaceuticals may prove to be one of the profession's most formidable challenges.

While the future of Keur Serigne Bi remains to be seen, ambulatory vendors continue to hawk their wares in the vicinity of Keur Serigne Bi and throughout Senegambia. The subregion has become the center of the trade in not only pharmaceuticals but also psychotropic drugs, and the trafficking of both is growing at staggering rates, helped by the porous borders and increasing instability of many countries along the Bight of Benin and the Windward Coast and in the Sahel. Drugs are shipped from Latin America to West Africa, where they enter networks that bring them to other parts of Africa as well as to Europe and Asia. The history of the traffic in psychotropic drugs is as rich as that of the traffic in pharmaceuticals. In the last decade, much research on this topic has been done, as academic and policy interest has grown. My next project will investigate drug trafficking in its legal and extralegal forms.

Conclusion

By the end of the twentieth century, Senegal's biomedical professionals had successfully adapted Western-derived ideas about healing and health care and made them their own. Biomedical training and practice was a lasting byproduct of France's colonial encounter with Senegal. Medicine based on bioscience reshaped approaches to the prevention and treatment of disease in this West African nation, and pharmacists have transformed ideas about what it means to offer healing techniques. While pharmacists face growing challenges from such factors as competing parallel markets, new pharmaceutical partners, and the proliferation of pharmacies, they continue to prove themselves resilient in the face of changes at the local and international levels.

The history of this transition saw locals initially reluctant to embrace European healing methods. It was a few decades before Africans became comfortable with biomedical healing approaches. The efficacy of biomedical treatment was continually challenged. In fact, many patients continued to simultaneously visit biomedical and traditional healers for treatment of illnesses and ailments. This practice of combining elements from different healing traditions continues. Today, health consumers also seek pharmaceuticals in both formal and informal sectors.

Although Western biomedicine would replace many networks of traditional healers, it enabled networks among African health providers, medical students, and professional communities to flourish. The professionalization of African health care providers trained in Western biomedicine transformed health care in the new nation of Senegal. Between 1918 and 1960, Africans who became doctors, nurses, midwives, and pharmacists were required to commit ten years to the colonial enterprise after earning their degrees. This lengthy service commitment, as well as patterns of discrimination, kept many from opening private practices during the colonial era. After independence, however, African professionals were eager to open private practices, because they offered more autonomy, more control over the conditions of work, and the possibility of higher income. In the late colonial and early postcolonial periods, pharmacies owned by Senegalese nationals replaced many of those owned by French immigrants.

As patterns of ownership changed, Senegalese women were also entering previously male-dominated pharmacy professions. Previously, women had worked in health care only as midwives and nurses. The change in attitude and in the admission policies of medical schools saw women become pharmacists, doctors, and dentists. As a result, between the 1950s and the 1970s, a group of pioneering women entered and gradually transformed pharmacy ownership in Senegal, as this study documents.

Women's professional development was also affected by the persistence of traditional values and attitudes. Senegal is a Muslim country, and its citizens adhere to a patriarchal tradition. Indeed, this book has shown how men and women delicately negotiated for recognition. In the early phases of female professionalism and pharmacy ownership, women surmounted gender and racial barriers by creating gender-based networks within a predominately male and significantly European-dominated sector. Women pharmacists exploited and transformed professional networks to gradually create a mixed-sex power base from which to enter the realm of professional leadership. Starting in the 1960s, women began to hold office in health care organizations. This achievement of recognition and status led them to play a dominant role in their profession's politics; it also inspired female pharmacy students and facilitated their entry into the profession. My research shows that by the 1980s, women had come to own a large percentage of pharmacies in Senegal, and by 2000, they owned 65 percent of all pharmacies in Dakar.

In the last two decades of the twentieth century, pharmacy owners—women and men—encountered new challenges, such as the devaluation of the currency, the unregulated proliferation of new pharmacies, and the burgeoning illegal trade in pharmaceuticals. These challenges led to economic instability, greater difficulty in managing pharmacies, and increased concerns for public health. Professional health care providers have begun to respond to these challenges by working with the government to better regulate illegal markets and to tighten lax regulations. Pharmacists have also begun to diversify their stock. They no longer only sell pharmaceuticals but are beginning to sell items found in American drugstores, such as cosmetics, toiletries, gifts, and in rare cases clothing. In addition, they have sought to remain relevant by better advertising their businesses in their neighborhoods and by improving customer service. Further, other health professionals are capitalizing on global networks and working with NGOs such as USAID on international projects.

Today banks, pharmaceutical wholesalers, and manufacturers readily do business with both men and women. Although foreign governments and agencies continue to work with African men on development projects in other sectors, women have cornered the pharmacy domain. Indeed, as pharmacists are often the primary deliverers of health care, this feminization of pharmacy in Senegal may lead to a greater inclusion of women in global policymaking. As this history has shown, once these industrious women enter the market, they utilize their capabilities to become prominent figures.

In the last decade, sub-Saharan Africa's public health sectors have moved in new directions. The pharmaceutical market is expanding faster in Africa than almost anywhere else in the world; recent estimates place it at more than US$10 billion per year, possibly reaching US$24 billion in 2014 and US$30 billion by 2016. This rapid growth has significant implications for pharmaceutical research, development, distribution, and marketing. Indeed, sub-Saharan Africa has become a part of the international medical industry complex. Like people in the rest of the world, Africans are also a part of the commercial drug marketing enterprise. As Africa plays a larger role in the global economy, health care plays a major role in its economy.

In addition, residents of the continent are facing a rise in affluence-related illnesses. African professionals in general have developed networks and improved their incomes, and some countries have relatively stable middle classes. But as incomes rise and citizens migrate in large numbers to urban centers, they encounter pollution, chemically enhanced foods, and high population density. Some of these changes, coupled with increasingly sedentary lifestyles, correlate to an increase in diseases such as diabetes, hypertension, and cancer. Finally, the rise in drug-resistant illnesses, especially some types of tuberculosis and malaria, is creating acute and major health crises both in Africa and beyond. In the case of tuberculosis, especially, contagion can easily cross national borders. As Africans travel more and the continent welcomes more tourists, there is always the possibility of an epidemic.

In this study, I have argued that pharmacists strategically navigated colonial and postcolonial realities to gain prominence as the key biomedical providers in postcolonial Senegal. It is my hope that scholars will continue to pursue new lines of inquiry as they study the intersections of public health, medical professionalization, gender, and entrepreneurship in sub-Saharan Africa. The role of pharmacists in Senegal is critical, as they are front-line medical providers. Historically these professionals have been the nexus between patients and new directions in public health. By consulting, diagnosing illness, and providing medical interventions, they play a more proactive role than many Western pharmacists. They also contribute to biomedical interventions by developing new pharmaceutical innovations in the laboratories. By collaborating with governmental and nongovernmental agencies on public health projects, they have made major contributions to the state of health in Senegal. We have much to learn from Senegalese pharmacists and their continued contributions to global health security.

Notes

Introduction

1. In this book, I usually use "pharmacist" and "pharmacy owner" synonymously. Unless I specify otherwise, they are the same. One must hold a pharmacy degree to own a pharmacy in Senegal. This is a book that focuses on the rise of a class of medical professionals and their evolution as entrepreneurial pharmacy owners. If a pharmacist does not own a pharmacy, I will note this in the text.

2. John Iliffe, *East African Doctors: A History of the Modern Profession* (Cambridge: Cambridge University Press, 1998); Adell Patton, *Physicians, Colonial Racism, and Diaspora in West Africa* (Gainesville: University Press of Florida, 1996); Pascale Barthélémy, "La professionnalisation des Africaines en AOF (1920–1960)," *Vingtième siècle, Revue d'histoire,* no. 75 (2002–2003): 36; Shula Marks, *Divided Sisterhood: Race, Class, and Gender in the South African Nursing Profession* (London: St. Martin's, 1994); Jane Turrittin, "Colonial Midwives and Modernizing Childbirth in French West Africa," in *Women in African Colonial Histories,* ed. Jean Allman, Susan Geiger, and Nakanyike Musisi (Bloomington: Indiana University Press, 2002), 71.

3. Didier Fassin, *Pouvoir et maladie en Afrique: Anthropologie sociale dans la banlieue de Dakar* (Paris: Presses universitaires de France, 1992); Diane Barthel, "The Rise of a Female Professional Elite: The Case of Senegal," *African Studies Review* 18, no. 3 (December 1975): 1–17; Stephen Addae, *History of Western Medicine in Ghana, 1880–1960* (Durham, N.C.: Durham Academic Press, 1997).

4. Informal economic activity is often not monitored or taxed by the government. It is also sometimes illegal. See Gracia Clark, *Onions Are My Husband: Survival and Accumulation by West African Market Women* (Chicago: University of Chicago Press, 1994); Judith Byfield, *The Bluest Hands: A Social and Economic History of Women Dyers in Abeokuta (Nigeria), 1890–1940* (Portsmouth, N.H.: Heinemann, 2002); Claire Robertson, *Trouble Showed the Way: Women, Men, and Trade in the Nairobi Area, 1890–1990* (Bloomington: Indiana University Press, 1997). On women in the formal economy, see Gloria Chuku, *Igbo Women and Economic Transformation in Southeastern Nigeria, 1900–1960* (New York: Routledge, 2005); Barthel, "The Rise of a Female Professional Elite"; Marks, *Divided Sisterhood;* Philomina E. Okeke-Ihejirika, *Negotiating Power and Privilege: Igbo Career Women in Contemporary Nigeria* (Athens: Ohio University Center for International Studies, 2004).

5. Myron Echenberg, *Black Death, White Medicine: Bubonic Plague and the Politics of Public Health in Colonial Senegal, 1914–1945* (Portsmouth, N.H.: Heinemann, 2002), 160.

6. Omar Ndoye, *Le n'döep: Transe thérapeuthique chez les Lébous du Sénégal* (Paris: L'Harmattan, 2010).

7. Anne-Marie Moulin, "Patriarchal Science: The Network of the Overseas Pasteur Institutes," in *Science and Empires: Historical Studies about Scientific Development and European Expansion,* ed. Patrick Petitjean, Catherine Jami, and Anne Marie Moulin (Dordrecht: Kluwer Academic Publishers, 1992), 303–22.

8. Christophe Bonneuil, *Des savants pour l'empire: La structuration des recherches scientifiques colonials au temps de "la mise en valeur des colonies françaises";* *1917–1945* (Paris: ORSTOM, 1991).

9. Aimée Houemavo, "Les médecins africains d'une élite coloniale," MA thesis, Université de Dakar, 1979.

10. Louis-Eugene-Benoît-Léon Couvy, *L'école de médecine indigène de l'Afrique occidentale française* (Dakar: Gouvernement général de l'Afrique occidentale française, 1930), 199. All translations of French texts and of interviews conducted in French are my own; I have sometimes retained French phrases for emphasis.

11. "L'éducation africaine," *Bulletin d'informations et de renseignements,* 15 August 1938, 303; "Arrêté: Portant organisation de l'École de médecine de l'Afrique occidental française," ANS 1H 24 (26).

12. Brahima Ouattara worked as a research assistant in tandem with me in 2008–2009. I gathered all of the other material alone.

13. Her letter was addressed to *chères consoeurs,* "dear sisterhood," indicating the prominent role played by female pharmacy owners. A few male pharmacists who read it commented that they found its language exclusionary.

14. *Tontines* are rotating credit associations that provide credit to entrepreneurs and family members. While many people rely on these as an alternative to formal credit assistance, others use them to supplement existing credit or income.

1. France's Biomedical Expansion

Epigraph quoted in René Dubos, *Pasteur and Modern Science* (Garden City, N.Y.: Doubleday, 1960), 145. Pasteur made the statement during a toast at a scientific conference in Milan in 1876.

1. Maghan Kéita, *A Political Economy of Health Care in Senegal* (Leiden: Brill, 2007), 58–59.

2. Toyin Falola and Matthew M. Heaton, eds., *Traditional and Modern Health Systems in Nigeria* (Trenton, N.J.: African World Press, 2006); Toyin Falola, *A Mouth Sweeter than Salt: An African Memoir* (Ann Arbor: University of Michigan Press, 2004); Nwando Achebe, *Farmers, Traders, Warriors, and Kings: Female*

Power in Northern Igboland, 1900–1960 (Portsmouth, N.H.: Heinemann, 2005);
P. Engelhard and L. Robineau, "La pharmacopée, composante de l'économie de la
santé au Sénégal," *Environnement africain,* occasional papers 59 (1981); Kéita, *A
Political Economy of Health Care in Senegal;* Susan Rasmussen, *Those Who Touch:
Tuareg Medicine Women in Anthropological Perspective* (Dekalb: Northern Illinois University Press, 2006); Joseph Kerharo, "La pharmacopée sénégalaise: Note
sur quelques traitements médicaux pratiqués par les Sarakolé du Cercle de Bakel,"
Bulletin et mémoires de la Faculté mixte de médecine et de pharmacie de Dakar, no.
12 (1964): 226–29.

3. Steven Feierman and John M. Janzen, eds., *The Social Basis of Health and
Healing in Africa* (Berkeley: University of California Press, 1992).

4. Kéita, *A Political Economy of Health Care in Senegal,* 63. For further reading, see Alice L. Conklin, *A Mission to Civilize: The Republican Idea of Empire in
France and West Africa, 1895–1930* (Palo Alto: Stanford University Press, 2000);
and Jean-Paul Bado, *Les conquêtes de la médecine moderne en Afrique* (Paris: Karthala, 2006).

5. Roy Porter, *The Greatest Benefit to Mankind: A Medical History of Humanity*
(New York: W. W. Norton, 1997), 113.

6. Saïbou Maïga, *Évolution de la pharmacie en Afrique occidentale française
(AOF), 1803–1960: Aspects législatifs et réglementaires* (Bamako, LINO Imprimerie
nouvelle, 2010), 31.

7. Steven Feierman, "Struggles for Control: The Social Roots of Health and
Healing in Modern Africa," *African Studies Review* 28, nos. 2–3 (1985): 74.

8. Aïssatou Moreau, interview by author, Dakar, 9 January 2001.

9. Kéita, *A Political Economy of Health Care in Senegal;* William Cohen, "Malaria and French Imperialism," *Journal of African History* 24, no. 1 (January 1983):
23–36; Philip D. Curtin, "Medical Knowledge and Urban Planning in Tropical
Africa," *American Historical Review* 90, no. 3 (June 1985): 594–613; Myron Echenberg, *Black Death, White Medicine: Bubonic Plague and the Politics of Public
Health in Senegal, 1914–1945* (Portsmouth, N.H.: Heinemann, 2002); Kalala Ngalamulume, "Keeping the City Totally Clean: Yellow Fever and the Politics of Prevention in Colonial Saint-Louis-du-Sénégal, 1850–1914," *Journal of African History* 45, no. 2 (July 2004): 183–202.

10. Pierre Pluchon, *Histoire des médecins et pharmaciens de marine et des colonies* (Paris: Privat, 1985), 422.

11. Alain Sinou, *Comptoirs et villes coloniales du Sénégal: Saint-Louis, Gorée,
Dakar* (Paris: Karthala, 1991), 141–43.

12. Angélique Diop, "Les débuts de l'action sanitaire de la France en AOF,
1895–1920: Le cas du Sénégal," in Charles Becker, Saliou M'baye, and Ibrahima
Thioub, *AOF: Réalités et héritages: Sociétés ouest-africaines et ordre colonial, 1895–
1960* (Dakar: Direction des archives du Sénégal, 1997), 2:1214.

13. Maïga, *Évolution de la pharmacie*, 46.

14. J. L. Oudart, "Les pharmaciens coloniaux," *Médecine tropicale* 65, no. 3 (2005): 263–72. In 1890, there were thirty-four colonial pharmacists; by 1954, the number had grown to 154.

15. Maïga, *Évolution de la pharmacie*, 56, 57.

16. Albert Calmette was one of France's most prominent colonial medical officials. In addition to his groundbreaking scientific developments, such as creating a vaccine for tuberculosis, he also set up the first overseas Pasteur Institute in Saigon in 1890.

17. Oudart, "Les pharmaciens coloniaux," 269.

18. Jean-François Le Blanc, interview by author, Paris, 11 January 2009.

19. Pierre Pluchon, "Action et recherches des figures," in Pluchon, *Histoire des médecins et pharmaciens,* 397. As head pharmacist, Busson helped to manage colonial medical personnel in French West Africa.

20. Anne Marie Moulin, "Patriarchal Science: The Network of the Overseas Pasteur Institutes," in *Science and Empires: Historical Studies about Scientific Development and European Expansion,* ed. Patrick Petitjean, Catherine Jami, and Anne Marie Moulin (Dordrecht: Kluwer Academic Publishers, 1992), 303–22; Christophe Bonneuil, *Des savants pour l'empire: La structuration des recherches scientifiques coloniales au temps de "la mise en valeur des colonies françaises"; 1917–1945* (Paris: ORSTOM, 1991).

21. Maïga, *Évolution de la pharmacie.*

22. Raymond Betts, "The Establishment of the Medina in Dakar, Senegal, 1914," *Africa: Journal of the International African Institute* 41, no. 2 (April 1971): 144.

23. Barthélémy Pascale, *Africaines et diplômées à l'époque coloniale, 1918–1957* (Rennes: Presses universitaires de Rennes, 2010), 24–25.

24. Gouverneur général de l'Afrique occidentale française, "Arrêté portant sur l'organisation de l'École de médecine de l'Afrique occidental française," ANS 1H 24 (26), 1–2.

25. Aimée Houemavo, "Les médecins africains d'une élite coloniale," MA thesis, Université de Dakar, 1979.

26. Aristide Le Dantec, "L'école de médecine indigène de Dakar," *Bulletin de la Société de pathologie exotique et de ses filiales* 13, no. 8 (1920): 623.

27. Jean François Le Blanc, interview by author, Paris, 11 January 2009.

28. John Iliffe, *East African Doctors: A History of the Modern Profession* (Cambridge: Cambridge University Press, 1998); Adell Patton, *Physicians, Colonial Racism, and Diaspora in West Africa* (Gainesville: University Press of Florida, 1996); Heather Bell, *Frontiers of Medicine in the Anglo-Egyptian Sudan, 1899–1940* (London: Oxford University Press, 1999). Bell finds that World War I was one of the factors urging the opening of a medical school in Sudan, as it was in French West Africa.

29. Mamadou Diouf, "The French Colonial Policy of Assimilation and the Civility of the Originaires of the Four Communes (Senegal): A Nineteenth Century Globalization Project," *Development and Change* 29, no. 4 (October 1998): 676.

30. Other territories controlled by France included Madagascar, Reunion, and the Seychelles.

31. Le Dantec, "L'école de médecine indigène," 625.

32. Ouezzin Coulibaly, "Sur l'éducation des femmes indigènes," *Éducation africaine,* nos. 99–100 (January–June 1938): 36. Similarly, in *Ambiguous Adventure* (Portsmouth, N.H.: Heinemann, 1972), Cheikh Amadou Kane highlights the dilemma that Senegalese parents faced in sending their children to French schools during the colonial years.

33. "Section des élèves sages-femmes," ANS 1H 24 (26).

34. Barthélémy, *Africaines et diplômées à l'époque coloniale,* 27.

35. Louis-Eugene-Benoît-Léon Couvy, *L'école de médecine indigène de l'Afrique occidentale française* (Dakar: Gouvernement général de l'Afrique occidentale française, 1930), 303.

36. Charles de Gaulle, "Décret du 11 août 1994," *Journal officiel de l'Afrique occidentale française,* December 1944, 813.

37. Le Dantec, "L'école de médecine indigène," 627.

38. "L'éducation africaine," *Bulletin d'informations et de renseignements,* 15 August 1938, 303.

39. Ibid., 305.

40. "Titre III: Élèves—études—examens," *Journal officiel de l'Afrique occidentale française,* 2 December 1944, 316.

41. Ibid., 814.

42. Colonel Garcin to Directeur général de l'intérieur, n.d., "Activités médicales de la Direction des affaires politique, 1945–1956," ANS 1H 24 (24).

43. Couvy, *L'école de médecine indigène,* 27.

44. "Rapport au President de la république," ANS 1H 7(1).

45. École de médecine et de pharmacie Jules Carde, "Promotion des élèves de 1922 à 1953," n.d., Archives de médecine et pharmacie, Université Cheikh Anta Diop, Dakar; École de médecine et de la pharmacie, "Rapport annuel, 1945–1946," Archives de médecine et pharmacie, Université Cheikh Anta Diop, Dakar. The latter report shows that four students were admitted in pharmacy that year.

46. Gouverneur général de l'Afrique occidentale française, "Arrêté—Portant sur l'organisation de l'École de médecine de l'Afrique occidental française," articles 18–20, ANS IH 24 (24).

47. Ibid., sections de médecine, pharmacie, et sages-femmes.

48. Alcantara, unpublished memoir in my possession, 82.

49. This business, now called Pharmacie Guigon, is perhaps the oldest operating pharmacy in Senegal, and is one of the oldest on the African continent. "Ar-

rêté no. 533: Autorisant Rito Alcantara à ouvrir une officine de pharmacie à Dakar, rue Gambetta," *Journal officiel du Sénégal* 2571 (1949): 89.

50. Alcantara memoir, 84.

51. Majhemout Diop, *Mémoires de luttes: Textes pour servir à l'histoire du Parti africain de l'indépendance* (Paris: Présence africaine, 2007), 25; Majhemout Diop, interview by author, Dakar, 8 May 2001.

52. Majhemout Diop, *Mémoires de luttes*, 30.

53. Aoua Kéita, *Femme d'Afrique: La vie d'Aoua Kéita racontée par elle-même* (Paris: Présence africaine, 1975), 23, 24, 169.

54. Birago Diop, *La plume raboutée* (Paris: Présence africaine, 1978), 52, 59, 76.

55. Siradiou Diallo, *Houphouët-Boigny: Le médecin, le planteur et le ministre (1900[?]–1960)* (Paris: Jeune Afrique livres, 1993), 41.

56. Other medical professionals, such as Félix Roland Moumié (Cameroon) and Issa and Felicia Basse (Senegal), followed similar trajectories.

57. "Bulletin d'information de l'AOF," *Journal officiel de l'Afrique occidentale française* 76, no. 16 (November 1950): 8, 9.

58. "Bulletin d'information de l'AOF," *Journal officiel de l'Afrique occidentale française* (1938): 199.

59. In follow-up interviews, a number of pharmacy owners were asked about their experience in Qur'anic school. Most said that they, like the majority of Senegalese children, had attended Qur'anic school in the years leading up to primary school. Many attended Qur'anic and primary schools concurrently. Some pharmacists, like Pape Amadou N'diaye, attended Qur'anic school into their teens.

60. See Anne-Marie Javouhey, *Correspondance, 1798–1851,* vol. 1 (Paris: Éditions du Cerf, 1994).

61. Archives mission de Dakar, *Annales religieuses de Dakar,* 26 April 1863, 361.

62. Bado, *Les conquêtes*, 38.

63. Michel Foucault, *Power* (New York: New Press, 1994), 137.

64. Ibid., 152–53.

65. Frantz Fanon, *The Wretched of the Earth,* trans. Constance Farrington (New York: Grove, 1963), 35.

66. Ibid., 53. On the psychological impact on the colonizer as well as the colonized, also see Albert Memmi, *Portrait du colonisé, précédé par Portrait du colonisateur,* translated as *The Colonizer and the Colonized* (New York: Beacon, 1991).

67. Similar ideas about blackness and dual identity were first published by the American scholar W. E. B. Du Bois in *The Souls of Black Folk* (Chicago: A. C. McClurg, 1903). Du Bois raises the idea of "double consciousness," in which men are always viewing themselves through the gaze of others.

68. Frantz Fanon, *Black Skin, White Masks,* trans. Charles L. Markmann (Paris: Éditions du Seuil, 1967, 89, 95.

69. David Macey, *Frantz Fanon: A Biography* (New York: Picador, 2000), 143.

70. Frantz Fanon, *A Dying Colonialism* (New York: Grove), 129–31.

71. Kéita, *Femme d'Afrique*, 95.

72. Maríama Bâ, interview by Alioune Touré Dia, *Amina*, November 1979, 12–14.

73. Echenberg, *Black Death, White Medicine*, 151.

74. Ibid.

75. Commandant de Cercle de Kajoor (Tivaouane) to Gouverneur du Sénégal, 12 May 1913, quoted in Kalala Ngalamulume, "City Growth, Health Problems, and Colonial Government Response: Saint-Louis (Senegal) from Mid-nineteenth Century to the First World War" (PhD diss., Michigan State University, 1996), 252.

2. Practicing Pharmacy

Epigraph from Antonin Fayemi, interview by Brahima Ouattara, Dakar, 16 November 2008.

1. Solange Diallo Decupper, interview by author, Dakar, 8 March 2001.

2. Gouverneur général de l'Afrique occidental française, Loi 54-48, 10 October 1955, Dakar, ANS 1H 24 (24).

3. Adolphe Touffait to Monsieur le Haut commissaire AOF, 11 August 1955, ANS 1H 7 (1).

4. Bernard Guigon, interview by author, Dakar, 4 May 2001; "Arrêté no. 533: Autorisant Rito Alcantara à ouvrir une officine de pharmacie à Dakar, rue Gambetta," *Journal officiel du Sénégal* 2571 (1949): 89; Rito Alcantara, interview by author, Dakar, 14 March 2001; École de médecine et de pharmacie Jules Carde, "Promotion des elèves de 1922 à 1953," Archives de médecine et pharmacie, Université Cheikh Anta Diop, Dakar, n.d. This latter document shows that two women graduated from the School of Pharmacy during this period: Maimouna Touré (1945) and Sara Coulibaly (1951). Many of the female enrollees did not complete their studies. One, Felicia Basse, completed her studies later and went on to open Pharmacie Cayor in Thiès, Senegal. See Majhemout Diop, interview by author, Dakar, 8 May 2001; N'deye Dieynaba Mbodj Fall, interview by author, Dakar, 21 August 2001.

5. Samir Amin, *Le monde des affaires sénégalaises* (Paris: Minuit, 1969), 156–57.

6. The date of his pharmacy's founding was significant to Alcantara, because it was his father's birthday. Rito Alcantara, interview by author, Dakar, 14 March 2001.

7. Ibid.

8. Ibid.

9. Ibid.

10. Majhemout Diop, interview by author, Dakar, 2001.

11. Majhemout Diop, *Mémoires de luttes: Textes pour servir à l'histoire du Parti africain de l'indépendance* (Paris: Présence africaine, 2007), 27–28.

12. The founding members of the PAI were African professionals and students committed to African political liberation and self-rule. The party incorporated ideals from scientific socialism as well as concepts and theories from African thought.

13. Diop married five times between the late 1950s and the 1980s; these unions produced twelve children. He died in Dakar on 27 January 2007 at age eighty-four.

14. Marie Laure Konate, interview by author, Dakar, 15 February 2001.

15. Antonin Fayemi, interview by Brahima Ouattara, Dakar, 16 November 2008.

16. Ibid.; Antonin Christian Bankolé Marie Fayemi, request to work at Laborex, dated 10 May 1983 and approved on 3 August 1983, Archives de l'Ordre national des pharmaciens, Dakar.

17. Hélène Akindes, interview by author, Dakar, 14 February 2001.

18. Pape Amadou N'diaye, interview by Brahima Ouattara, Dakar, 27 October 2008.

19. N'deye Toutane Thiam Ngom, interviews by author, Dakar, 11, March 2001 and by Brahima Ouattara, Dakar, 14 January 2009.

20. N'deye Toutane Thiam Ngom, interview by author, Dakar, 11 March 2001.

21. Annette Seck N'diaye, interview by author, Dakar, 20 December 2000.

22. Senegal, Ministère de la femme, de l'enfant et de la famille, *Femmes sénégalaises à l'horizon 2015* (Dakar: Ministère de la femme, de l'enfant et de la famille, 1993), 83.

23. École de médecine et de pharmacie, "Nombre d'étudiants enscrits, 1983–1991," Archives de médecine et pharmacie, Université Cheikh Anta Diop, Dakar.

24. Senegal, Ministère de la femme, de l'enfant et de la famille, *Femmes sénégalaises à l'horizon 2015,* 83.

25. Faculté de médecine et de pharmacie, Service de la scolarité et des examens, "Statistiques des étudiants inscrits," Université Cheikh Anta Diop, 1992.

3. Women Own Pharmacies Too

Epigraph from Aïssatou Moreau, interview by author, Dakar, 9 January 2001.

1. Gracia Clark, *Onions Are My Husband: Survival and Accumulation by West African Market Women* (Chicago: University of Chicago Press, 1994); Judith A. Byfield, *The Bluest Hands: A Social and Economic History of Women Dyers in Abeokuta (Nigeria), 1890–1940* (Portsmouth, N.H.: Heinemann, 2002); Claire Robertson, *Trouble Showed the Way: Women, Men, and Trade in the Nairobi Area, 1890–1990* (Bloomington: Indiana University Press, 1997); Mary Johnson Osirim,

Enterprising Women in Urban Zimbabwe: Gender, Microbusiness, and Globalization (Washington, D.C.: Woodrow Wilson Center Press, 2009).

2. Gloria Chuku, *Igbo Women and Economic Transformation in Southeastern Nigeria, 1900–1960* (New York: Routledge, 2005); Diane Barthel, "The Rise of a Female Professional Elite: The Case of Senegal," *African Studies Review* 18, no. 3 (December 1975): 1–17; Shula Marks, *Divided Sisterhood: Race, Class, and Gender in the South African Nursing Profession* (London: St. Martin's, 1994); Philomena E. Okeke-Ihejirika, *Negotiating Power and Privilege: Igbo Career Women in Contemporary Nigeria* (Athens: Ohio University Center for International Studies, 2004).

3. Jean Allman, Susan Geiger, and Nakanyike Musisi, eds., *Women in African Colonial Histories* (Bloomington: Indiana University Press, 2002); Anne Hugon, ed., *Histoire des femmes en situation coloniale: Afrique et Asie, XXe siècle* (Paris: Karthala, 2004); Odile Goerg, ed., *Perspectives historiques sur le genre en Afrique* (Paris: L'Harmattan, 2007); Dorothy L. Hodgson and Sheryl A. McCurdy, eds., *"Wicked" Women and the Reconfiguration of Gender in Africa* (Portsmouth, N.H.: Heinemann, 2001).

4. In the 1970s and 1980s, see George Brooks, "The *Signares* of Saint-Louis and Gorée: Women Entrepreneurs in Eighteenth-Century Senegal," in *Women in Africa: Studies in Social and Economic Change,* ed. Nancy Hafkin and Edna Bay (Stanford: Stanford University Press, 1976), 19–44; Colette Le Cour Grandmaison, "Activités économiques des femmes dakaroises," *Africa: Journal of the International African Institute* 39 (1969): 138–52; Alice Hamer, "Diola Women and Migration: A Case Study," in *The Uprooted of the Western Sahel: Migrants' Quest for Cash in the Senegambia,* ed. Lucie Gallistel Colvin et al. (New York: Praeger, 1981): 59–80; Régine Bonnardel, "Saint-Louis du Sénégal: Le règne des femmes dans les petites activités," in *Processus d'urbanisation en Afrique,* ed. Catherine Coquery-Vidrovitch (Paris: L'Harmattan, 1988), 2:130–40. For later investigations of these topics, see Fatou Sarr, *L'entrepreneuriat féminin au Sénégal: La transformation des rapports de pouvoirs* (Paris: L'Harmattan, 1998); Wilmetta J. Toliver-Diallo, "'The Woman Who Was More than a Man': Making Aline Sitoe Diatta into a National Heroine in Senegal," *Canadian Journal of African Studies* 39, no. 2 (2005): 338–60; Donna Perry, "Wolof Women, Economic Liberalization, and the Crisis of Masculinity in Rural Senegal," *Ethnology* 44, no. 3 (summer 2005): 207–26; Coumba Mar Gadio and Cathy A. Rakowski, "Farmers' Changing Roles in Thieudeme, Senegal: The Impact of Local and Global Factors on Three Generations of Women," *Gender and Society* 13, no. 6 (December 1999): 733–57.

5. Michel Foucault uses the phrase "economy of health" to mean an advanced stage of development of biomedical institutions and of the consumption of biomedicine. "The Birth of Social Medicine," in *Power,* ed. James D. Faubion, vol. 3 of *The Essential Works of Foucault, 1954–1984* (New York: New Press, 2000): 135.

6. Emmanuel Grégoire and Pascal Labazée, eds., *Grands commerçants d'Afrique de l'ouest: Logiques et pratiques d'une groupe d'hommes d'affaires contem-*

porains (Paris: Karthala, 1993); Boubacar Barry and Leonhard Harding, *Commerce et commerçants en Afrique de l'Ouest*, vol. 1, *Le Sénégal* (Paris: L'Harmattan, 1993); Stephen Ellis and Yves-A. Fauré, *Entreprises et entrepreneurs africains* (Paris: Karthala, 1995); Laurence Marfaing and Mariam Sow, *Les opérateurs économiques au Sénégal: Entre le formel et l'informel (1930-1996)* (Paris: Karthala, 1999).

7. Pascale Barthélémy, "La professionalisation des africaines en AOF (1920–1960)," *Vingtième siècle, Revue d'histoire*, no. 75 (July–September 2002): 36.

8. "Arrêté no. 729 autorisant Madame Pétrau ouvrir une pharmacie à Diourbel," *Journal officiel du Sénégal* 2521 (3 March 1948): 150; "Arrêté no. 905 autorisant Mademoiselle Chanteau, Yvonne ouvrir une officine à Dakar," *Journal officiel du Sénégal* 2521 (13 March 1948): 150. Mrs. Pétrau's first name is not available in archival records.

9. "Decision no. 5098 autorisant Mme Martin, née Durand (Jacqueline, Marie-Louise) pharmacienne à Dakar, à remplacer M. Guigon," *Journal officiel du Sénégal* 2658 (12 September 1950): 761.

10. École de médecine et de pharmacie Jules Carde, "Promotion des élèves de 1922 à 1953," Archives de médecine et pharmacie, Université Cheikh Anta Diop, Dakar, n.d.

11. Basse was active in the PAI, with Majhemout Diop (also a pharmacist); her husband, Issa Basse (a dental surgeon); Félix Moumié (a doctor); and other Francophone African professionals.

12. N'deye Dieynaba Mbodj Fall, interview by author, Dakar, 21 August 2001.

13. École de médecine et pharmacie, *Rapport annuel* (1945–1946).

14. Senegal, Ministère de la femme, de l'enfant et de la famille, *Femmes sénégalaises a l'horizon 2015* (Dakar: Ministère de la femme, de l'enfant et de la famille, 1993), 83.

15. N'deye Dieynaba Mbodj Fall, interview by author, Dakar, 21 August 2001.

16. Ministère de la santé, "Arrêté ministerial no. 8031," *Journal officiel du Sénégal* 3459 (1961): 969.

17. Samir Amin, *Le monde des affaires sénégalaises* (Paris: Minuit, 1969), 156–57. Similarly, Rito Alcantara established a pharmacy in 1949 at the periphery of the central city.

18. Solange Diallo Decupper, interview by author, Dakar, 8 March 2001.

19. Rita O'Brien, *White Society in Black Africa: The French of Senegal* (Evanston, Ill.: Northwestern University Press, 1972).

20. Solange Diallo Decupper, interview by author, Dakar, 8 March 2001.

21. Other women who held office between the late 1970s and the 1990s include Maïmouna Diop, N'deye Toutane Thiam Ngom, Annette Seck N'diaye, and Khady Bao.

22. Marie Emilienne Tavares, interview by author, Dakar, 10 January 2001.

23. A memo in the Archives de l'Ordre national des pharmaciens, Dakar, Senegal, dated 19 January 1975, chronicles this election. In the first round of voting, Fall and Alcantara had four votes each, and Kandji had one. In the second round, Fall received five votes and Alcantara received four.

24. Anta Sar, interview by Brahima Ouattara, Dakar, 17 December 2008.

25. Maïmouna Diop, e-mail to author, 21 December 2010.

26. Unpublished record of sale, "Convention de cession d'une officine," between Bao and Ghandour, 31 July 1998, Dakar; Khady Bao, interview by author, Dakar, 30 March 2001.

27. Senegalese women wanting to become pharmacists increasingly pursue degrees abroad, most often in France, Canada, and the United States. Some return to Senegal, but more and more of them choose to stay in the country where they earned their degree, usually working for large pharmaceutical chains.

28. Nafissatou Bao Mbaye, interview by author, Dakar, 22 March 2001.

29. Bineta Dia, interview by author, Dakar, 18 January 2001.

30. Hawoly Wane Sy, interview by author, Dakar, 5 February 2001.

31. Aby Kane Diallo, interview by author, Dakar, 30 March 2001.

32. World Health Organization, "Le secteur pharmaceutique privé commercial au Sénégal: Dynamique de développement et effet sur l'accès aux médicaments essentiels" (Geneva: World Health Organization, 1997), 17.

33. Ministère de la santé, Décrets nos. 8-243 and 8-244.

34. Chandra Mohanty, Ann Russo, and Lourdes Torres, eds., *Third World Women and the Politics of Feminism* (Bloomington: Indiana University Press, 1991).

35. Fatou Sow, "Les initiatives féministes au Sénégal: Une réponse à la crise?" *Africa développement (Actes du Colloque sur l'état et la société au Sénégal: Crises et dynamiques sociales)* 18, no. 3 (1993): 89–115; Ellen Bortei-Doku Aryeetey and Ernest Aryeetey, *Operation, Utilization and Change in Rotating Susu Savings in Ghana* (Legon: Institute of Statistical, Social and Economic Research, University of Ghana, 1996).

36. Marième N'diaye, interview by author, Dakar, 23 April 2001.

37. Maïmouna Diop, e-mail to author, 21 December 2010.

38. Marie Emilienne Tavares, interview by author, Dakar, 10 January 2001.

4. House and Street

Epigraph from Maïmouna N'diaye Niang, interview by author, Dakar, 11 February 2001.

1. For further discussion, see Fiona McLaughlin, "Haalpulaar Identity as a Response to Wolofization," *African Languages and Cultures* 8, no. 2 (January 1995): 153–68.

2. Among them were Marie Emilienne Bâ and Jeanne Vidal Sall.

3. Marie Emilienne Bâ, interview by author, Dakar, 9 March 2001.

4. Hawoly Wane Sy, interview by author, Dakar, 5 March 2001. The demands of balancing private and professional life became too daunting for Sy, and she sold her pharmacy a few years after this interview.

5. Touty Diack Dia, interview by Brahima Ouattara, Thiaroye, Senegal, 29 October 2008.

6. Khady Bengeloum Diallo, interview by Brahima Ouattara, Dakar, 30 October 2008.

7. Annette Seck N'diaye, interview by author, Dakar, 20 December 2000.

8. Mariane Coly, interview by author, Dakar, 28 March 2001.

9. Solange Diallo Decupper, interview by Brahima Ouattara, Dakar, 17 December 2008.

10. Anta Sar, interview by Brahima Ouattara, Dakar, 17 December 2008.

11. Elisabeth McMahon and Corrie Decker, "Wives or Workers? Negotiating the Social Contract between Female Teachers and the Colonial State in Zanzibar," *Journal of Women's History* 21, no. 2 (summer 2009): 39–61. Also see the broad literature on women's power, honor, and respectability in Latin American history, including work by Susan Besse, Sueann Caulfield, Muriel Nazzari, and Irene Silverblatt.

12. Tabaski is Eid al-Kebir, a Muslim holiday associated with Abraham's sacrifice. Korité is Eid al-Fitr, the holiday that marks the end of Ramadan.

13. Aïssatou Moreau, interview by author, Dakar, 9 January 2001.

14. Sarah Mirza and Margaret Strobel, eds., *Three Swahili Women: Life Histories from Mombasa, Kenya* (Bloomington: Indiana University Press, 1999); Belinda Bozzoli, with Mmantho Nkotsoe, *Women of Phokeng: Consciousness, Life Strategy and Migrancy in South Africa, 1900–1983* (Portsmouth, N.H.: Heinemann, 1991); Maríama Bâ, *So Long a Letter* (Portsmouth, N.H.: Heinemann, 1981).

15. Senegalese scholars have provided well-developed accounts of women's social and familial obligations, particularly in regard to marriage. See, for example, Fatou Binetou Dial, *Mariage et divorce à Dakar: Itinéraires féminins* (Paris: Karthala, 2008); Abdoulaye Bara Diop, *La famille Wolof: Tradition et changement* (Paris: Karthala, 1985).

16. Dial, *Mariage et divorce à Dakar*, 29.

17. Senegalese couples can choose between monogamy, restricted polygyny, and unrestricted polygyny. Dial unpacks the four types of polygyny as categorized by Phillipe Antoine and Jeanne Nanitelamaio: "imposed polygyny," "polygyny of the poor," "ostentatious polygyny," and "*polygamie de retour.*"

18. Loi no. 73–62, 29 December 1962.

19. Ordre national des pharmaciens, *Recueil de textes de base régissant la pharmacie au Sénégal* (Dakar: Ordre national des pharmaciens, 1999), 8.

20. Helmut Kloos et al., "The Utilization of Pharmacies and Pharmaceutical Drugs in Addis Ababa, Ethiopia," *Social Science and Medicine* 22, no. 6 (1986): 653–72.

21. "Demander une autorisation d'ouverture d'une officine privée de pharmacie: Liste Pieces à fournir pour ouvrir une officine," Archives de l'Ordre national des pharmaciens, Dakar.

22. These memos are discussed in Ordre national des pharmaciens, memo to Ministre de la santé, requesting authorization for Dr. Touré to work at Parke Davis (1985), Archives de l'Ordre National des pharmaciens, Dakar.

23. Request by Antonin Fayemi to work at Laborex made on 10 May 1983 and approved on 3 August 1983, Archives de l'Ordre national des pharmaciens, Dakar.

24. Babacar Fall, *Ajustement structurel et emploi au Sénégal* (Paris: Karthala, 1997), xiii. Between 1981 and 1991, Senegal received 4.3 percent of all international aid going to the African continent. This is significant for one small country on a continent with more than fifty others.

25. Ordre national des pharmaciens, "Inter-l'ordre circulaire sur le devaluation," 25 March 1994, Archives de l'Ordre national des pharmaciens, Dakar.

26. Marie Emilienne Bâ, interview by author, Dakar, 9 March 2001.

27. Ministère de la santé, "Arrêté no. 11265 du 19 août 1992 fixant le nombre de pharmacien-assistants chiffres d'affaires . . . 100,000,000 CFA," and "Arrêté no. 9089 du 14 décembre 1998 fixant le nombre de pharmaciens-assistants dans les officines," Archives de l'Ordre national des pharmaciens, Dakar.

28. Record of sale, "Convention de cession d'une officine," between Khady Bao and Mohamed Ghandour, buyer of her pharmacy, Archives de l'Ordre national des pharmaciens, Dakar.

29. Marc Sankalé, *Médecins et action sanitaire en Afrique noire* (Paris: Présence africaine, 1969), 335; Ministère du développement industriel, "Perspective de l'industrie pharmaceutique au Sénégal: Problèmes et solutions" (Dakar, 1970); P. Engelhard and L. Robineau, "La pharmacopée, composante de l'économie de la santé au Sénégal," *Environnement africain,* occasional papers 59 (1981): 60–63; Donna A. Patterson, "Maïmouna Diop: Improving Senegal's Public Health Sector through Pharmaceutical Equivalence," Heroes and Great Ideas Column, *Journal of Health Care for the Poor and Underserved* 24, no. 1 (2013): 11.

30. Interview with N'deye Toutane Thiam Ngom, interview by author, Dakar, 11 March 2001.

31. Khady Bengeloum Diallo, interview by Brahima Ouattara, Dakar, 30 October 2008.

32. Counterfeit drugs are produced by manufacturers that do not hold a patent for them. These drugs may or may not contain the same ingredients as the true drug.

33. Annette Seck N'diaye, interview by author, Dakar, 20 December 2000.

34. Meredith Turshen, "Reprivatizing Pharmaceutical Supplies," in *Privatizing Health Services in Africa* (New Brunswick, N.J.: Rutgers University Press, 1999), 97, 199.

35. Daniel Callahan and Angela Wasunna, *Medicine and the Market: Equity v. Choice.* (Baltimore: Johns Hopkins University Press, 2006), 167, 179.

36. Diana Senghor, "Marché des dupes," *Vivre autrement,* no. 2 (1985): 31.

37. Ministère de la santé, Décret no. 81-244, "Fixant provisoirement le nombre et la répartition des pharmacies," Dakar, 13 March 1981.

38. Engelhard and Robineau, "La pharmacopée," 88.

39. Ministère de la santé, Décret no. 81-244, Dakar, 13 March 1981.

40. Ministère de la santé to Ordre national des pharmaciens, 16 April 1987, Archives de l'Ordre national des pharmaciens, Dakar.

41. Ordre national des pharmaciens, "Compte rendu de l'audience avec monsieur le President de la République," 21 August 1981, Archives de l'Ordre national des pharmaciens, Dakar. François Gaye, a former officeholder in the Pharmacy Syndicate, was the owner of Pharmacie Thiaroye-sur-Mer at that time.

42. Ordre national des pharmaciens to Minister Marie Mbodji Sarr, 25 July 1989, Archives de l'Ordre national des pharmaciens, Dakar.

43. *Journal officiel du République du Sénégal,* décret no. 93-1060, "Fixant les critères et la répartition des officines de pharmacie" (1995): 370.

44. Arrêté no. 7865, "Fixant provisoirement le nombre et la répartition des officines de pharmacie en AOF," 10 October 1955, Archives de l'Ordre national des pharmaciens, Dakar.

45. Abdoulahat Mangane, a Ministry of Health officer, and I computed these figures from unpublished Ministry of Health documents on 9 August 2001; Annette Seck N'diaye, interview by author, Dakar, 20 December 2000.

46. Ministre Marie Mbodji Sarr, letter to Ordre national des pharmaciens, 30 June 1990, Archives de l'Ordre national des pharmaciens, Dakar.

47. A series of letters and memos in my possession chronicle Tharcisse Nkulikiyinfura's appeals, which began in 1990. Particularly interesting are the letters from him to N'deye Dieynaba Fall, dated 24 April 1996, and to Ousmane Ngom, an official at the Ministry of Health, dated 25 June 1996.

48. Mariane Coly, interview by author, Dakar, 28 March 2001; Aïssatou Moreau, interview by author, Dakar, 10 January 2001; Hawoly Wane Sy, interview by author, Dakar, 5 February 2001; Hélène Akindes, interview by author, Dakar, 14 February 2001.

49. Mame Awa Guèye Diop, interview by author, Dakar, 28 August 2001.

50. Marie Laure Konate, interview by author, Dakar, 15 February 2001.

51. Khady Bengeloum Diallo, interview by Brahima Ouattara, Dakar, 30 October 2008.

52. Oumy Ndoye Fall, interview by author, Dakar, 23 April 2001.

53. Faculté de médecine et de pharmacie de Dakar, "L'évolutions [des nombres d'étudiants]," 11 November 1991, Archives de médecine et pharmacie, Université Cheikh Anta Diop, Dakar.

54. Rokhaya Sylla Guéye, interview by author, Dakar, 17 January 2001; Bineta Dia, interview by author, Dakar, 18 January 2001; Marie Laure Konate, interview by author, Dakar, 28 August 2001.

55. Sokhna Boye Soumare, interview by author, Dakar, 1 May 2001; Mariane Coly, interview by author, Dakar, 28 March 2001; Khady Bengeloum Diallo, interview by Brahima Ouattara, Dakar, 30 October 2008.

5. Pharmaceutical Trafficking in Colonial and Postcolonial Senegal

Epigraph from Jean-François Bayart, Stephen Ellis, and Beatrice Hibou, introduction to *The Criminalization of the State in Africa* (Bloomington: Indiana University Press, 1999), xvi.

1. Harold L. Wilensky, "The Professionalization of Everyone?" *American Journal of Sociology* 70, no. 2 (September 1964): 156.

2. Willem van Schendel, "Spaces of Engagement: How Borderlands, Illegal Flows, and Territorial States Interlock," in *Illicit Flows and Criminal Things: States, Borders, and the Other Side of Globalization,* ed. Willem van Schendel and Itty Abraham (Bloomington: Indiana University Press, 2005), 48.

3. Fatou Mbengue, "Le marché parallèle dans le département de Dakar et Pikine au Sénégal" (PhD diss., Université Cheikh Anta Diop, 1993); Cheikh Tidiane Diaw, "La vente illicite des médicaments dans les marchés et rues au Sénégal: Enquêtes effectuées dans les regions de Dakar, Kaolack et Diourbel" (PhD diss., Université Cheikh Anta Diop, 1992); Charles Albert Panka, "La vente illicite des médicaments au Cameroun: Exemple de la ville de Douala" (PhD diss., Université Cheikh Anta Diop, 1994); and Vincent Hamel, "La vente illicite de médicaments dans les pays en développement: Analyse de l'émergence d'un itinéraire thérapeutique à part entière, situé en parallèle du recours classique aux structures officielles de santé" (PhD diss., Université Claude Bernard Lyon I, 2006).

4. Bayart, Ellis, and Hibou, *The Criminalization of the State in Africa,* 16.

5. Jean Comaroff and John Comaroff, *Law and Disorder in the Postcolony* (Chicago: University of Chicago Press, 2006).

6. "Globalisation et illicite en Afrique," *Politique africaine,* no. 93 (March 2004).

7. Lori Leonard, "Where There Is No State: Household Strategies for the Management of Illness in Chad," *Social Science and Medicine* 61, no. 1 (July 2005): 229–43; Helmut Kloos et al., "The Utilization of Pharmacies and Pharmaceutical Drugs in Addis Ababa, Ethiopia," *Social Science and Medicine* 22, no. 6 (1986)

653–72; Sjaak van der Geest, "Self-Care and the Informal Sale of Drugs in South Cameroon," *Social Science and Medicine* 25, no. 3 (1987): 293–305.

8. Axel Klein, "Trapped in the Traffick: Growing Problems of Drug Consumption in Lagos," *Journal of Modern African Studies* 32, no. 4 (December 1994): 657–77; Emmanuel Akyeampong, "Diaspora and Drug Trafficking in West Africa: A Case Study of Ghana," *African Affairs* 104, no. 416 (July 2005): 429–47; Centre tricontinental, *Drogues et narco-trafic: Le point de vue du Sud* (Paris: L'Harmattan, 1996); Stephen Ellis, "West Africa's International Drug Trade," *African Affairs* 108, no. 431 (April 2009): 171–96

9. Didier Fassin, "La vente illicite des médicaments au Sénégal: Economies 'parallèles,' État et société," *Politique africaine,* no. 23 (October 1986): 123–30; Didier Fassin, *Pouvoir et maladie en Afrique: Anthropologie sociale dans la banlieue de Dakar* (Paris: Presses universitaires de France, 1992); Donna A. Patterson, "Local Borders and Global Flows: Senegal's Illegal Pharmaceutical Trade," *Harvard Africa Policy Journal* 6 (April 2010): 21–33.

10. Didier Fassin, "Du clandestine à l'officieux: Les réseaux de vente illicite des médicaments au Sénégal," *Cahiers d'études africaines* 25, no. 98 (1985): 161–77.

11. Counterfeit drugs also move along these networks, particularly from Nigeria and China but also from India. Like the parallel trade in pharmaceuticals, this is a growing problem. Counterfeit drugs are being increasingly discovered not only in Asia and Africa but also in Europe and North America. Some are chemically exact copies of the real drug, while others contain chalk, talcum powder, or other inert ingredients.

12. Patterson, "Local Borders and Global Flows," 24–26.

13. David Anderson et al., *The Khat Controversy: Stimulating the Debate on Drugs* (Oxford: Berg, 2007); Ezekiel Gebissa, *Leaf of Allah: Khat and Agricultural Transformation in Harerge, Ethiopia, 1875–1991* (Athens: Ohio University Press, 2004); Gernot Klantschnig, "The Politics of Law Enforcement in Nigeria: Lessons from the War on Drugs," *Journal of Modern African Studies* 47, no. 4 (December 2009): 529–49.

14. Dr. Garcin to Haut-commissaire en AOF, 23 August 1950, ANS 1 H 48 (144).

15. Pharmacien commandant Perrotto to Pharmacien chef de la Côte d'Ivoire, 1950, ANS 1 H 48 (144).

16. Postscript to Dr. Garcin's letter to Directeur général de l'intérieur sur . . . le trafic illicite en AOF, 23 August 1950, ANS 1 H 48 (144).

17. Gouverneur de la Côte d'Ivoire to Haut-commissaire de la République française, Gouverneur général de l'AOF, 12 August 1950, ANS 1 H 48 (144).

18. Gouverneur de la Côte d'Ivoire to Haut-commissaire de la République française, 15 October 1950, ANS 1 H 48 (144).

19. H. Gazagnon, Chef de la Sureté, to Inspecteur général de la Sureté en AOF sur le trafic produits pharmaceutiques, 27 March 1951, ANS 1 H 48 (144).

20. Ibid., pp. 2–4.

21. Eric Ross, "Touba, A Spiritual Metropolis in the Modern World," *Canadian Journal of African Studies* 29, no. 2 (1995): 229–59.

22. Cheikh Anta Mbacke Babou, "Amadu Bamba and the Founding of the Muridiyya: The History of a Muslim Brotherhood in Senegal, 1853–1913" (PhD diss., Michigan State University, 2002), 287.

23. For example, see Mamadou Diouf, "The Senegalese Murid Trade Diaspora and the Making of a Vernacular Cosmopolitanism," *Public Culture* 12, no. 3 (fall 2000): 679–702.

24. Ibid.

25. Achille Mbembe, "Africa's Frontiers in Flux," *Le monde diplomatique,* 12 November 1999, 23.

26. Christian Coulon and Donal B. Cruise O'Brien, "Senegal," in *Contemporary West African States,* ed. Donal Cruise O'Brien, John Dunn, and Richard Rathbone (Cambridge, Cambridge University Press, 1989), 156.

27. This hospital was completed in 2003 through donations from far-flung Mouride merchants. It is jointly operated by the state and the Mouride brotherhood. See Ellen Foley and Cheikh Anta Babou, "Diaspora, Faith, and Science: Building a Mouride Hospital in Senegal," *African Affairs* 110, no. 438 (January 2011): 75–95.

28. Ordre national des pharmaciens, "Securité et accessibilité du médicament en Afrique," paper presented at the Forum pharmaceutique international de Dakar, 18–21 June 2001.

29. Fassin, *Pouvoir et maladie en Afrique;* Mavelout Dieng, "Problematique de marché illicite de médicament," unpublished report for the Association des jeunes pharmaciens sénégalais, Dakar, 2002; Patterson, "Local Borders and Global Flows."

30. Fassin, *Pouvoir et maladie en Afrique,* 90.

31. Diaw, "La vente illicite des médicaments," 50.

32. Paul Stoller, *Money Has No Smell: The Africanization of New York City* (Chicago: University of Chicago Press, 2002), 5.

33. "A.," interview by author, 14 February 2000, Dakar. In this chapter I use initials and not names, because of the sensitive nature of the topic.

34. Mbengue, "Le marché parallèle"; Diaw, "La vente illicite des médicaments."

35. "S.," interview by author, 11 January 2001. Traditionally, a Baol was a subject of the former Baol kingdom, which included contemporary Touba in its environs. The terms "Baol-Baol" and "Modou-Modou" now refer to migrating Mouride traders.

36. "N.," interview by author, 20 April 2001; "S.," interview by author, 11 January 2001; "D.," interview by author, 18 January 2001.

37. Dieng, "Problematique de marché illicite de médicament."

38. Jean Marc Guimier et al., "Pourquoi le prix des médicaments est élevé dans les pays d'Afrique subsaharienne: Analyse de la structure des prix; L'exemple du Sénégal," *Cahiers santé* 15, no. 1 (January–March 2005): 44.

39. "N." interviews by author, 20 April and 20 December 2000.

40. Ordre national des pharmaciens, "Securité et accessibilité du médicament en Afrique."

41. Minutes of "Illicit Sale of Drugs in Parallel Markets," a meeting at the Forum pharmaceutique international de Dakar, 21 June 2001.

42. Idrissa Sané, "Mamadou Ndiadé, président de l'ordre des pharmaciens: Le marché noir est une menace pour le secteur de la pharmacie," *Le soleil,* 16 October 2006.

43. Fara Diaw, "Commerce illicite de médicaments: Un trafic juteux et nocif," *Le soleil,* 17 November 2001; Jean-Marc Guimier and Danielle Candau, *Étude sur l'accessibilité au médicament: Rapport definitif* (Dakar: Ministère de la santé publique, Syndicat national de l'industrie pharmaceutique, 2001); Patterson, "Local Borders and Global Flows."

44. Fassin, "Du clandestine à l'officieux," 170.

45. Owen Dyer, "New Report on Corruption in Health," *Bulletin of the World Health Organization,* 84, no. 2 (February 2006), 84–85.

46. Robert Cockburn et al., "The Global Threat of Counterfeit Drugs: Why Industry and Government Must Communicate the Dangers," *PLoS Medicine* 2, no. 4 (April 2005); Tim Phillips, *Knockoff: The Deadly Trade in Counterfeit Goods* (London: Kogan Page, 2005).

Selected Bibliography

Informants

Ahoomey, Florence Apovo
Akindes, Hélène
Alcantara, Rito
Bâ, Amadou
Bâ, Marie Emilienne
Badiane, Emmanuel
Bao, Khady
Bassene, Emmanuel
Brelot, Fabienne Alcantara
Cissé, Malick
Coly, Mariane
Decupper, Solange Diallo
Dia, Bineta
Dia, Fatoumata
Dia, Oumar
Dia, Touty Diack
Diallo, Aby Kane
Diallo, Aminata
Diallo, Khady Bengeloum
Dièye, Khadim
Diop, Aissatou Guèye
Diop, Maïmouna
Diop, Majhemout
Diop, Mame Awa Guèye
Diouf, El Hajj
Fall, N'deye Dieynaba Mbodj
Fall, Oumy Ndoye

Fayemi, Antonin
Gaye, Thérèze Diop
Guéye, Aïssatou
Guéye, Rokhaya Sylla
Guigon, Bernard
Kfoury, Georges
Konate, Marie Laure
Le Blanc, Jean François
Lô, Issa
Mangane, Abdoulahat
Mbaye, Nafissatou Bao
Moreau, Aïssatou
Ndiadé, Mamadou
N'diaye, Aby
N'diaye, Badara Louis
N'diaye, Dorothée
N'diaye, Marième
N'diaye, Pape Amadou
N'diaye, Sokhna Diagne
Ngom, N'deye Toutane Thiam
Niang, Amath
Niang, Maïmouna N'diaye
Sall, Jeanne Vidal
Samb, Khady Fall
Sar, Anta
Seck, Colette M. H.
Seck N'diaye, Annette
Slyva, Alexandre J. Th.
Soumare, Sokhna Boye
Sow, Fatou Dia
Sy, Hawoly Wane
Sylla, Mame Penda Fofana
Tavares, Marie Emilienne
Thiaw, Abdoulaye
Touré, Aissatou Diouf

Archives and Collections

Archives de l'Ordre national des pharmaciens, Dakar, Senegal
Archives du Ministère de la santé et direction de la pharmacie, Dakar, Senegal
Archives de médecine et pharmacie, Université Cheikh Anta Diop, Dakar, Senegal

Archives nationales de France, Section outre-mer, Afrique occidentale française, Aix-en-Provence, France
Archives nationales du Sénégal, Dakar, Senegal
Archives de l'Afrique occidental française, Dakar, Senegal

Books and Articles

Achebe, Nwando. *Farmers, Traders, Warriors, and Kings: Female Power and Authority in Northern Igboland, 1900–1960.* Portsmouth, N.H.: Heinemann, 2005.

Akyeampong, Emmanuel. "Diaspora and Drug Trafficking in West Africa: A Case Study of Ghana." *African Affairs* 104, no. 416 (July 2005): 429–47.

Allman, Jean, Susan Geiger, and Nakanyike Musisi, eds. *Women in African Colonial Histories.* Bloomington: Indiana University Press, 2002.

Ambler, Charles. "Alcohol, Racial Segregation and Popular Politics in Northern Rhodesia." *Journal of African History,* no. 31 (July 1990): 295–313.

Amin, Samir. *Le monde des affaires sénégalais.* Paris: Minuit, 1969.

Antoine, Phillipe, and Jeanne Nanitelamaio. *Peut-on échapper à la polygamie à Dakar?* Paris: CEPED, 1995.

Aryeetey, Ellen Bortei-Doku, and Ernest Aryeetey. *Operation, Utilization and Change in Rotating Susu Savings in Ghana.* Legon: Institute of Statistical, Social and Economic Research, University of Ghana, 1996.

Bâ, Maríama. *So Long a Letter.* Portsmouth, N.H.: Heinemann, 1981.

———. Interview by Alioune Touré Dia. *Amina,* November 1979, 12–14.

Babou, Cheikh Anta Mbacke. "Amadu Bamba and the Founding of the Muridiyya: The History of a Muslim Brotherhood in Senegal, 1853–1913." PhD diss., Michigan State University, 2002.

Bado, Jean-Paul. *Les conquêtes de la médecine moderne en Afrique.* Paris: Karthala, 2006.

Barrows, Leland C. "Faidherbe and Senegal: A Critical Discussion." *African Studies Review* 19, no. 1 (April 1976): 95–117.

Barthel, Diane. "The Rise of a Female Professional Elite: The Case of Senegal." *African Studies Review* 18, no. 3 (December 1975): 1–17.

———. "Women's Educational Experience under Colonialism: Toward a Diachronic Model." *Signs* 11, no. 1 (fall 1985): 137–54.

Barthélémy, Pascale. *Africaines et diplômées à l'époque coloniale, 1918–1957.* Rennes: Presses universitaires de Rennes, 2010.

———. "La formation des Africaines à l'École normale d'institutrices de l'AOF de 1938 à 1958: Instruction ou éducation?" *Cahiers d'études africaines* 43, nos. 169–70 (2003): 371–88.

———. "La professionalisation des africaines en AOF (1920–1960)." *Vingtième siècle, Revue d'histoire,* no. 75 (July–September 2002): 35–46.

Bayart, Jean-François. "Le crime transnational et la formation de l'État." *Politique africaine,* no. 93 (March 2004): 93–103.

Bayart, Jean-François, Stephen Ellis, and Beatrice Hibou. *The Criminalization of the State in Africa.* Bloomington: Indiana University Press, 1999.

Beck, Linda J. "Reining in the Marabouts? Democratization and Local Governance in Senegal." *African Affairs* 100, no. 401 (October 2001): 601–21.

Becker, Charles, and René Collignon. "Épidémies et médecine coloniale en Afrique de l'Ouest." *Cahiers d'études et de recherches francophones: Santé* 8, no. 6 (December 1998): 411–16.

Becker, Charles, et al. "Recueil de textes législatifs et réglementaires relatifs à la santé: Éléments d'un code de la santé publique au Sénégal." Unpublished paper, 2001.

Becker, Charles, Saliou M'baye, and Ibrahima Thioub. *AOF: Réalités et héritages; Sociétés ouest-africaines et ordre colonial, 1895–1960.* 2 vols. Dakar: Direction des archives du Sénégal, 1997.

Bell, Heather. *Frontiers of Medicine in the Anglo-Egyptian Sudan, 1899–1940.* Oxford: Oxford University Press, 1999.

Berger, Iris. "African Women's History: Themes and Perspectives." *Journal of Colonialism and Colonial History* 4, no. 1 (spring 2003).

Betts, Raymond. "The Establishment of the Medina in Dakar, Senegal, 1914." *Africa: Journal of the International African Institute* 41, no. 2 (April 1971): 143–52.

Blassingame, John. *The Slave Community: Plantation Life in the Antebellum South.* Oxford: Oxford University Press, 1972.

Bonnardel, Régine. "Saint-Louis du Sénégal: Le règne des femmes dans les petites activités." In *Processus d'urbanisation en Afrique,* edited by Catherine Coquery-Vidrovitch, 2:130–40. Paris: L'Harmattan, 1988.

Bonneuil, Christophe. *Des savants pour l'empire: La structuration des recherches scientifiques coloniales au temps de "la mise en valeur des colonies françaises"; 1917–1945.* Paris: ORSTOM, 1991.

Botte, Roger. "Vers un État illégal-légal?" *Politique africaine,* no. 93 (March 2004): 7–20.

Bouche, Denise. "L'enseignement dans les territoires français de l'Afrique occidentale de 1817 à 1920." PhD diss., Université de Lille III, 2 vols., 1975.

Bozzoli, Belinda, with Mmantho Nkotsoe. *Women of Phokeng: Consciousness, Life Strategy and Migrancy in South Africa, 1900–1983.* Portsmouth, N.H.: Heinemann, 1991.

Brooks, George E., Jr. "The *Signares* of Saint-Louis and Gorée: Women Entrepreneurs in Eighteenth-Century Senegal." In *Women in Africa: Studies in Social and Economic Change,* edited by Nancy J. Hafkin and Edna G. Bay, 19–44. Stanford: Stanford University Press, 1976.

"Bulletin d'information de l'AOF." *Journal officiel de l'Afrique occidentale française*, no. 76 (16 November 1950): 8.

Byfield, Judith A. *The Bluest Hands: A Social and Economic History of Women Dyers in Abeokuta (Nigeria), 1890–1940.* Portsmouth, N.H.: Heinemann, 2002.

Callahan, Daniel, and Angela A. Wasunna. *Medicine and the Market: Equity v. Choice.* Baltimore: Johns Hopkins University Press, 2006.

Chuku, Gloria. *Igbo Women and Economic Transformation in Southeastern Nigeria, 1900–1960.* New York: Routledge, 2005.

Clark, Gracia. *Onions Are My Husband: Survival and Accumulation by West African Market Women.* Chicago: University of Chicago Press, 1994.

Cohen, William B. "Malaria and French Imperialism." *Journal of African History* 24, no. 1 (January 1983): 23–36.

Comaroff, Jean. "The Diseased Heart of Africa: Medicine, Colonialism, and the Black Body." In *Knowledge, Power, and Practice: The Anthropology of Medicine and Everyday Life,* edited by Shirley Lindenbaum and Margaret Lock, 305–29. Berkeley: University of California Press, 1993.

Comaroff, John, and Jean Comaroff. *Ethnography and the Historical Imagination.* Boulder: Westview, 1992.

Comaroff, Jean, and John Comaroff, eds. *Law and Disorder in the Postcolony.* Chicago: University of Chicago Press, 2006.

Conklin, Alice L. *A Mission to Civilize: The Republican Idea of Empire in France and West Africa, 1895–1930.* Stanford: Stanford University Press, 2000.

Cooper, Barbara M. *Marriage in Maradi: Gender and Culture in a Hausa Society in Niger, 1900–1989.* Portsmouth, N.H.: Heinemann, 1997.

Cornwall, Andrea, ed. *Readings in Gender in Africa.* Bloomington: Indiana University Press, 2005.

Coulibaly, Ouezzin. "Sur l'éducation des femmes indigènes." *Éducation africaine,* nos. 99–100 (January–June 1938): 33–36.

Coulon, Christian, and Donal B. Cruise O'Brien. "Senegal." In *Contemporary West African States,* edited by Donal B. Cruise O'Brien, John Dunn, and Richard Rathbone, 145–64. Cambridge: Cambridge University Press, 1989.

Courtwright, David T. *Forces of Habit: Drugs and the Making of the Modern World.* Cambridge, Mass.: Harvard University Press, 2001.

Couvy, Louis-Eugene-Benoît-Léon. *L'école de médecine indigène de l'Afrique occidentale française.* Dakar: Gouvernement général de l'Afrique occidentale française, 1930.

Crowder, Michael. *West Africa under Colonial Rule.* Evanston, Ill.: Northwestern University Press, 1968.

Curtin, Philip D. "Medical Knowledge and Urban Planning in Tropical Africa." *American Historical Review* 90, no. 3 (June 1985): 594–613.

Dial, Fatou Binetou. *Mariage et divorce à Dakar: Itinéraires féminins.* Paris: Karthala, 2008.

Diallo, Nafissatou. *A Dakar Childhood.* Translated by Dorothy S. Blair. London: Longman, 1982.

Diallo, Siradiou. *Houphouët-Boigny: Le médecin, le planteur et le ministre (1900[?]–1960).* Paris: Jeune Afrique livres, 1993.

Diaw, Cheikh Tidiane. "La vente illicite des médicaments dans les marchés et rues au Sénégal: Enquêtes effectuées dans les regions de Dakar, Kaolack et Diourbel." PhD diss., Université Cheikh Anta Diop, 1992.

Diaw, Fara. "Mamadou Ndiadé, president de l'ordre des pharmaciens: 'Le marché noir est une menace pour le secteur de la pharmacie.'" *Le soleil,* October 16, 2006.

Dieng, Mavelout. "Problematique de marché illicite de médicament." Unpublished report for the Association des jeunes pharmaciens sénégalaises (AJPS), Dakar, Senegal, 2002.

Diop, Abdoulaye Bara. *La famille Wolof: Tradition et changement.* Paris: Karthala, 1985.

Diop, Alioune. "History of a Black Schoolboy." *Éducation africaine* 76 (July–Sept) 1931: 25–29. Translated by Geoffrey Coats in "From Whence We Come: Alioune Diop and Saint-Louis, Senegal," *Research in African Literatures* 28, no. 4 (winter 1997): 206–19.

Diop, Angélique. "Les débuts de l'action sanitaire de la France en AOF, 1895–1920: Le cas du Sénégal." In Becker, M'baye, and Thioub, *AOF: Réalités et heritages,* 2:1212–27. Dakar: Direction des archives de Sénégal, 1997.

Diop, Birago. *La plume raboutée.* Paris: Présence africaine, 1978.

Diop, Maïmouna. *Mayite Equivalence.* Dakar: PUB, 2010.

Diop, Majhemout. *Mémoires de luttes: Textes pour servir à l'histoire du Parti africain de l'indépendance.* Paris: Présence africaine, 2007.

Diop, Momar-Coumba. "Les affaires mourides à Dakar." *Politique africaine,* no. 4 (December 1981): 90–100.

Diop, Pape Momar. "L'enseignement de la fille indigène en AOF, 1903–1958." In Becker, M'baye, and Thioub, *AOF: Réalités et heritages,* 2:1081–96. Dakar: Direction des archives de Sénégal, 1997.

Diouf, Mamadou. "The French Colonial Policy of Assimilation and the Civility of the Originaires of the Four Communes (Senegal): A Nineteenth Century Globalization Project." *Development and Change* 29, no. 4 (October 1998): 671–96.

Du Bois, W. E. B. *The Souls of Black Folk.* Chicago: A. C. McClurg, 1903.

Dubos, René. *Pasteur and Modern Science.* Garden City, N.Y.: Doubleday, 1960.

Echenberg, Myron. *Black Death, White Medicine: Bubonic Plague and the Politics of Public Heath in Colonial Senegal, 1914–1945.* Portsmouth, N.H.: Heinemann, 2002.

"L'éducation africaine." *Bulletin d'informations et de renseignements,* August 15, 1938, 303.

Ellis, Stephen. "West Africa's International Drug Trade." *African Affairs* 108, no. 431 (April 2009): 171–96.

Ellis, Stephen, and Yves-A. Fauré. *Entreprises et entrepreneurs africains.* Paris: Karthala, 1995.

Engelhard, P., and L. Robineau. "La pharmacopée, composante de l'économie de la santé au Sénégal." *Environnement africain.* Occasional papers 59 (1981).

Evans, Martin. "From Colonialism to Post-colonialism: The French Empire since Napoleon." In *French History since Napoleon,* edited by Martin S. Alexander, 391–415. Oxford: Oxford University Press, 1999.

Faidherbe, Louis Léon César. *Le Sénégal: La France dans l'Afrique occidentale.* Paris: Hachette, 1889.

Fainzaing, Sylvie, and Odile Journet. *La femme de mon mari: Étude ethnologique du mariage polygamique en Afrique et en France.* Paris: L'Harmattan, 1988.

Fall, Babacar. *Ajustement structurel et emploi au Sénégal.* Paris: Karthala, 1997.

Falola, Toyin. *A Mouth Sweeter than Salt: An African Memoir.* Ann Arbor: University of Michigan Press, 2004.

Falola, Toyin, and Matthew M. Heaton, eds. *Traditional and Modern Health Systems in Nigeria.* Trenton, N.J.: African World Press, 2006.

Fanon, Frantz. *Black Skin, White Masks.* Translated by Richard Philcox. New York: Grove, 2008.

——. *A Dying Colonialism.* New York: Grove, 1994.

——. *The Wretched of the Earth.* Translated by Constance Farrington. New York: Grove, 1963.

Fassin, Didier. *Les enjeux politiques de la santé: Études sénégalaises, équatoriennes et françaises.* Paris: Karthala, 2000.

——. *Pouvoir et maladie en Afrique: Anthropologie sociale dans la banlieue de Dakar.* Paris: Presses universitaires de France, 1992.

Feierman, Steven, and John M. Janzen, eds. *The Social Basis of Health and Healing in Africa.* Berkeley: University of California Press, 1992.

Flint, Karen E. *Healing Traditions: African Medicine, Cultural Exchange, and Competition in South Africa, 1820–1948.* Athens: Ohio University Press, 2008.

Foley, Ellen E. *Your Pocket Is What Cures You: The Politics of Health in Senegal.* New Brunswick: Rutgers University Press, 2010.

France. *Outre-Mer, 1959: Tableau économique et social des états et territoires d'Outre-Mer.* Paris: Presses universitaires, 1960.

Gadio, Coumba Mar, and Cathy A. Rakowski. "Farmers' Changing Roles in Thieudeme, Senegal: The Impact of Local and Global Factors on Three Generations of Women." *Gender and Society* 13, no. 6 (December 1999): 733–57.

Gaulle, Charles de. "Décret du 11 août 1994." *Journal officiel de l'Afrique occidentale française,* December 1944, 813.

Gebissa, Ezekiel. *Leaf of Allah: Khat and Agricultural Transformation in Harerge, Ethiopia, 1875–1991.* Athens: Ohio University Press, 2004.

Gilbert, Leah. "Dispensing Doctors and Prescribing Pharmacists: A South African Perspective." *Social Science and Medicine* 46, no. 1 (January 1998): 83–95.

———. "To Diagnose, Prescribe and Dispense: Whose Right Is It? The Ongoing Struggle between Pharmacy and Medicine in South Africa." *Current Sociology* 49, no. 3 (May 2001): 97–118.

Goerg, Odile. "Femmes africaines et pratique historique en France." *Politique africaine,* no. 72 (December 1998): 130–44.

Gomez, Michael A. *Exchanging Our Country Marks: The Transformation of African Identities in the Colonial and Antebellum South.* Chapel Hill: University of North Carolina Press, 1998.

Grandmaison, Colette Le Cour. *Femmes dakaroises: Rôles traditionnels féminins et urbanisation.* Annales de l'Université d'Abidjan, series F, ethnosociology. Abidjan: Université d'Abidjan, 1972.

Grégoire, Emmanuel, and Pascal Labazée, eds. *Grands commerçants d'Afrique de l'Ouest: Logiques et pratiques d'une groupe d'hommes d'affaires contemporains.* Paris: Karthala, 1993.

Gueye, S. "Vente illicite de médicaments: Les pharmaciens poursuivent le combat." *Le soleil,* 23 October 2003.

Guimier, Jean-Marc, and Danielle Candau. *Étude sur l'accessibilité au médicament: Rapport definitif.* Dakar: Ministère de la santé publique, Syndicat national de l'industrie pharmaceutique, 2001.

Hall, Gwendolyn Midlo. *Slavery and African Ethnicities in the Americas: Restoring the Links.* Chapel Hill: University of North Carolina Press, 2005.

Hamel, Vincent. "La vente illicite de médicaments dans les pays en développement: Analyse de l'émergence d'un itinéraire thérapeutique à part entière, situé en parallèle du recours classique aux structures officielles de santé." PhD diss., Université Claude Bernard Lyon I, 2006.

Hanson, John H. *Migration, Jihad, and Muslim Authority in West Africa: The Futanke Colonies in Karta.* Bloomington: Indiana University Press, 1996.

Hay, Margaret Jean. "Queens, Prostitutes, and Peasants: Historical Perspectives on African Women, 1971–1986." In "Current Research on African Women," special issue, *Canadian Journal of African Studies* 22, no. 3 (1988): 431–47.

Headrick, Rita. *Colonialism, Health, and Illness in French Equatorial Africa, 1885–1935.* Atlanta: African Studies Association Press, 1994.

Hine, Darlene Clark. *Black Women in White: Racial Conflict and Cooperation in the Nursing Profession, 1890–1950.* Bloomington: Indiana University Press, 1989.

Hodgson, Dorothy L., and Sheryl A. McCurdy, eds. *"Wicked" Women and the Re-configuration of Gender in Africa*. Portsmouth, N.H.: Heinemann, 2001.

Holloway, Joseph E., ed. *Africanisms in American Culture*. Bloomington: Indiana University Press, 1990.

Houemavo, Aimée. "Les médecins africains d'une élite coloniale." MA thesis, Université de Dakar, 1979.

Huff, Toby E. *The Rise of Early Modern Science: Islam, China, and the West*. 2nd ed. New York: Cambridge University Press, 2003.

Hugon, Anne, ed. *Histoire des femmes en situation coloniale: Afrique et Asie, XXe siècle*. Paris: Karthala, 2004.

Hunt, Nancy Rose. *A Colonial Lexicon: Of Birth Ritual, Medicalization, and Mobility in the Congo*. Durham, N.C.: Duke University Press, 1999.

———. "Placing African Women's History and Locating Gender." *Social History* 14, no. 3 (October 1989): 359–79.

Iliffe, John. *East African Doctors: A History of the Modern Profession*. Cambridge: Cambridge University Press, 1998.

Jalloh, Alusine. *African Entrepreneurship: Muslim Fula Merchants in Sierra Leone*. Athens: Ohio University Center for International Studies, 1999.

Javouhey, Anne-Marie. *Correspondance, 1798–1851*. Vol. 1. Paris: Éditions du Cerf, 1994.

Johnson, Wesley G. "The Impact of the Senegalese Elite upon the French, 1900–1940." In *Double Impact: France and Africa in the Age of Imperialism*, edited by G. Wesley Johnson, 155–78. Westport, Conn.: Greenwood, 1985.

Jones, Hilary. *The Métis of Senegal: Urban Life and Politics in French West Africa*. Bloomington: Indiana University Press, 2013.

Julien, Eileen. *African Novels and the Question of Orality*. Bloomington: Indiana University Press, 1992.

Kéita, Aoua. *Femme d'Afrique: La vie d'Aoua Kéita racontée par elle-même*. Paris: Présence africaine, 1975.

Keita, Maghan. *A Political Economy of Health Care in Senegal*. Leiden: Brill, 2007.

———. "The Political Economy of Health Care in Senegal: The Integration of Traditional and Modern Medicine Revisited." *Journal of Asian and African Studies* 31, nos. 3–4 (July 1996): 145–61.

Kerharo, Joseph. "La pharmacopée sénégalaise: Note sur quelques traitements médicaux pratiqués par les Sarakolé du Cercle de Bakel." *Bulletin et mémoires de la Faculté mixte de médecine et de pharmacie de Dakar*, no. 12 (1964): 226–29.

———. *La pharmacopée sénégalaise traditionelle: Plantes, médicinales, et toxiques*. Paris: Éditions Vigot frères, 1974.

Klantschnig, Gernot. "The Politics of Law Enforcement in Nigeria: Lessons from the War on Drugs." *Journal of Modern African Studies* 47, no. 4 (December 2009): 529–49.

Klein, Axel. "Trapped in the Traffick: Growing Problems of Drug Consumption in Lagos." *Journal of Modern African Studies* 32, no. 4 (December 1994): 657–77.

Kloos, Helmut, et al. "The Utilization of Pharmacies and Pharmaceutical Drugs in Addis Ababa, Ethiopia." *Social Science and Medicine 22,* no. 6 (1986): 653–72.

Le Dantec, Aristide. "L'école de médecine indigène de Dakar." *Bulletin de la Société de pathologie exotique et de ses filiales* 13, no. 8 (1920): 623–38.

Lom, Mika. "Médicaments: La défiance des pharmaciens." *Sud hebdo,* 16 April 1992.

Macey, David. *Frantz Fanon: A Biography.* New York: Picador, 2000.

Maïga, Saïbou. *Évolution de la pharmacie en Afrique occidentale française (AOF), 1803–1960: Aspects législatifs et réglementaires.* Bamako: LINO Imprimerie nouvelle, 2010.

Manning, Patrick. *Francophone Sub-Saharan Africa, 1880–1995.* Cambridge: Cambridge University Press, 1988.

Marfaing, Laurence, and Mariam Sow. *Les opérateurs économiques au Sénégal: Entre le formel et l'informel (1930–1996).* Paris: Karthala, 1999.

Marks, Shula. *Divided Sisterhood: Race, Class, and Gender in the South African Nursing Profession.* London: St. Martin's, 1994.

Martin, Phyllis M. "Celebrating the Ordinary: Church, Empire, and Gender in the Life of Mère Marie-Michelle Dédié (Senegal, Congo, 1882–1931)." *Gender and History* 16, no. 2 (August 2004): 289–317.

Masquelier, Adeline. "Beyond the Dispensary's Prosperous Façade: Imagining the State in Rural Niger." *Public Culture* 13, no. 2 (spring 2001): 267–92.

Mbembe, Achille. "Migration of Peoples, Disintegration of States: Africa's Frontiers in Flux." *Le monde diplomatique,* November 1999.

Mbengue, Fatou. "Le marché parallèle dans le département de Dakar et Pikine au Sénégal." PhD diss., Université Cheikh Anta Diop, 1993.

Mbow, Penda. "Les femmes, l'Islam, et les associations religieuses au Sénégal: Le dynamisme des femmes en milieu urbain." In *Transforming Female Identities: Women's Organizational Forms in West Africa,* edited by Eva Evers Rosander, 148–59. Uppsala: Nordiska Afrikainstitutet, 2000.

McLaughlin, Fiona. "Haalpulaar Identity as a Response to Wolofization." *African Languages and Cultures* 8, no. 2 (January 1995): 153–68.

McMahon, Elisabeth, and Corrie Decker. "Wives or Workers? Negotiating the Social Contract between Female Teachers and the Colonial State in Zanzibar." *Journal of Women's History* 21, no. 2 (summer 2009): 39–61.

McNee, Lisa. *Selfish Gifts: Senegalese Women's Autobiographical Discourses.* Albany: State University of New York Press, 2000.

Memmi, Albert. *The Colonizer and the Colonized.* Translated by Howard Greenfeld. Boston: Beacon, 1991.

Mirza, Sarah, and Margaret Strobel, eds. *Three Swahili Women: Life Histories from Mombasa, Kenya.* Bloomington: Indiana University Press, 1989.

Mohanty, Chandra, Ann Russo, and Lourdes Torres, eds. *Third World Women and the Politics of Feminism.* Bloomington: Indiana University Press, 1991.

Moulin, Anne Marie. "Patriarchal Science: The Network of the Overseas Pasteur Institutes." In *Science and Empires: Historical Studies about Scientific Development and European Expansion,* edited by Patrick Petitjean, Catherine Jami, and Anne Marie Moulin, 303–22. Dordrecht: Kluwer Academic Publishers, 1992.

Ngalamulume, Kalala. "City Growth, Health Problems, and Colonial Government Response: Saint-Louis (Senegal) from Mid-nineteenth Century to the First World War." PhD diss., Michigan State University, 1996.

———. *Colonial Pathologies, Environment, and Western Medicine in Saint-Louis-du-Senegal, 1867–1920.* New York: Peter Lang, 2012.

———. "Keeping the City Totally Clean: Yellow Fever and the Politics of Prevention in Colonial Saint-Louis-du-Sénégal, 1850–1914." *Journal of African History* 45, no. 2 (July 2004): 183–202.

Okeke-Ihejirika, Philomina E. *Negotiating Power and Privilege: Igbo Career Women in Contemporary Nigeria.* Athens: Ohio University Center for International Studies, 2004.

Ordre national des pharmaciens. *Securité et accessibilité du médicament en Afrique.* Dakar: Forum pharmaceutical international de Dakar, June 2001.

———. *Recueil de textes de base régissant la pharmacie au Sénégal.* Dakar: Ordre national des pharmaciens, 1999.

Oudart, J. L. "Les pharmaciens coloniaux." *Médecine tropicale* 65, no. 3 (2005): 263–72.

Panka, Charles Albert. "La vente illicite des médicaments au Cameroun: Exemple de la ville de Douala." PhD diss., Université Cheikh Anta Diop, 1994.

Patterson, Donna A. "Expanding Professional Horizons: Female Pharmacists in Twentieth-Century Dakar, Senegal." PhD diss., Indiana University, 2008.

———. "Local Borders and Global Flows: Senegal's Illegal Pharmaceutical Trade." *Harvard Africa Policy Journal* 6 (2010): 21–33.

———. "Women and Economic Change in Senegal." Unclassified report for the United States embassy in Senegal. 19 August 1998.

———. "Women Pharmacists in Twentieth-Century Senegal: Examining Access to Education and Property in West Africa." *Journal of Women's History* 24, no. 1 (spring 2012): 111–37.

Patton, Adell. *Physicians, Colonial Racism, and Diaspora in West Africa.* Gainesville: University Press of Florida, 1996.

Paulme, Denise, ed. *Women of Tropical Africa.* Berkley: University of California Press, 1960.

Pluchon, Pierre. *Histoire des médecins et pharmaciens de marine et des colonies.* Paris: Privat, 1985.

Porter, Roy. *The Greatest Benefit to Mankind: A Medical History of Humanity.* New York: W. W. Norton, 1997.

Raboteau, Albert J. *Slave Religion: The "Invisible Institution" in the Antebellum South.* New York: Oxford University Press, 1978.

Rasmussen, Susan J. *Those Who Touch: Tuareg Medicine Women in Anthropological Perspective.* Dekalb: Northern Illinois University Press, 2006.

Robertson, Claire. "A Growing Dilemma: Women and Change in African Primary Education, 1950–1980." *Journal of Eastern African Research and Development* 15 (1985): 17–35.

———. *Sharing the Same Bowl: A Socioeconomic History of Women and Class in Accra, Ghana.* Ann Arbor: University of Michigan Press, 1990.

———. *Trouble Showed the Way: Women, Men, and Trade in the Nairobi Area, 1890–1990.* Bloomington: Indiana University Press, 1997.

Robinson, David. "France as a Muslim Power in West Africa." *Africa Today,* nos. 3–4 (summer–fall 1999): 105–27.

Ross, Eric. "Touba: A Spiritual Metropolis in the Modern World." *Canadian Journal of African Studies* 29, no. 2 (1995): 229–59.

Sabatier, Peggy R. "'Elite' Education in French West Africa: The Era of Limits, 1903–1945." *International Journal of African Historical Studies* 11, no. 2 (1978): 247–66.

Sankalé, Marc. *Médecins et action sanitaire en Afrique noire.* Paris: Présence africaine, 1969.

Sankalé, Marc, and Pierre Pène. *Dossiers africains: Médecine sociale au Sénégal.* Dakar: Afrique-documents, 1960.

Sarr, Fatou. *L'entrepreneuriat féminin au Sénégal: La transformation des rapports de pouvoirs.* Paris: L'Harmattan, 1998.

Scott, Joan Wallach. *Gender and the Politics of History.* New York: Columbia University Press, 1988.

Senegal. Ministère de la femme, de l'enfant et de la famille. *Femmes sénégalaises a l'horizon 2015.* Dakar: Ministère de la femme, de l'enfant et de la famille, 1993.

Senghor, Diana. "Marché des dupes." *Vivre autrement,* no. 2 (1985): 21–34.

Senghor, Léopold Sédar. "Some Thoughts on Africa: A Continent in Development." Address at Chatman House, 25 October 1961. Reprinted in *International Affairs* (Royal Institute of International Affairs) 38, no. 2 (April 1962): 189–95.

Sinou, Alain. *Comptoirs et villes coloniales du Sénégal: Saint-Louis, Gorée, Dakar.* Paris: Karthala, 1991.

Sow, Bassirou. "Une profession à assainir." *Sud quotidien,* 20 August 1995.

Sow, Fatou. "Les initiatives féministes au Sénégal: Une réponse à la crise?" *Africa développement (Actes du Colloque sur l'état et la société au Sénégal: Crises et dynamiques sociales)* 18, no. 3 (1993): 89–115.

Suret-Canale, Jean. *French Colonialism in Tropical Africa, 1900–1945.* Translated by Till Gottheiner. New York: Pica, 1971.

Turrittin, Jane. "Colonial Midwives and Modernizing Childbirth in French West Africa." In Allman, Geiger, and Musisi, *Women in African Colonial Histories,* 71–95. Bloomington: Indiana University Press, 2002.

Turshen, Meredith. "Reprivatizing Pharmaceutical Supplies." In *Privatizing Health Services in Africa,* 97–113. New Brunswick, N.J.: Rutgers University Press, 1999.

van Schendel, Willem. "Spaces of Engagement: How Borderlands, Illegal Flows, and Territorial States Interlock." In *Illicit Flows and Criminal Things: States, Borders, and the Other Side of Globalization,* edited by Willem van Schendel and Itty Abraham, 38–68. Bloomington: Indiana University Press, 2005.

Vaughn, Megan. *Curing Their Ills: Colonial Power and African Illness.* Stanford: Stanford University Press, 1991.

Vidal, Laurent. *Les professionels de santé en Afrique de l'Ouest: Entre savoirs et pratiques; Paludisme, tuberculose, et prévention au Sénégal et en Côte d'Ivoire.* Paris: L'Harmattan, 2005.

Ware, Rudolph. "Njàngaan: The Daily Regime of Qur'ânic Students in Twentieth-Century Senegal." *International Journal of African Historical Studies* 37, no. 3 (2004): 515–38.

Weiss, Holger, ed. *Social Welfare in Muslim Societies in Africa.* Uppsala: Nordiska Afrikainstitutet, 2002.

Werner, Jean-François. *Marges, sexe, et drogues à Dakar: Enquête ethnographique.* Paris: Karthala, 1993.

White, Luise. *The Comforts of Home: Prostitution in Colonial Nairobi.* Chicago: University of Chicago Press, 1990.

White, Luise, Stephan F. Miescher, and David William Cohen, eds. *African Words, African Voices: Critical Practices in Oral History.* Bloomington: Indiana University Press, 2001.

World Health Organization. "Le secteur pharmaceutique privé commercial au Sénégal: Dynamique de développement et effet sur l'accès aux médicaments essentiels." Geneva: World Health Organization, 1997.

———. *WHO Traditional Medicine Strategy, 2002–2005.* Geneva: World Health Organization, 2002.

Yansané, A. Y. "The Impact of France on Education in West Africa." In *Double Impact: France and Africa in the Age of Imperialism,* edited by G. Wesley Johnson, 345–62. Westport, Conn.: Greenwood, 1985.

Index

"economy of health," 61, 135n5
education, 3, 23, 31–33, 37, 50, 94, 113; medical, 7, 8, 13, 20, 21, 22–31, 33–34, 38, 42, 46, 50, 52, 53–54, 60, 63–64, 66, 70, 83, 98, 123; women, 11, 23–24, 28–29, 37, 53–54, 60, 64, 66, 72, 75
Ellis, Stephen, 97, 99
entrepreneurship, 1, 3, 11, 12, 60, 61–66, 73, 74, 84, 108, 125
epidemics, 7–8, 15, 16, 18, 20–21, 25, 34, 125
Ethiopia, 82
ethnicity, 11, 14, 15, 32, 75, 95
évolués, 7
extralegal pharmaceutical trade, 51, 88, 96, 99, 101, 102, 104, 105, 106, 108–109, 114, 121

Fall, N'deye Dieynaba Mbodj, 1–2, 3, 9, 52, 63, 66, 67–68, 84
Fall, Oumy Ndoye, 94
family, 11, 24, 29, 37, 49, 51, 62, 69, 70, 74, 75–80, 113, 116
Fanon, Frantz, 34–36, 38; *Black Skin, White Masks,* 34, 35; *A Dying Colonialism,* 34, 36
Fassin, Didier, 100, 109, 119
Fayemi, Antonin, 40, 48–49, 52, 56, 83
Fayemi, Pierre, 28, 48, 49
Feierman, Steven, 16
Femme d'Afrique (Kéita), 36
Foucault, Michel, 33–34, 135n5
Four Communes of Senegal, 7, 18, 23
France: colonial education policy, 31–33; colonial health policy, 7, 16, 17–31, 38, 46, 63; colonialism, 38, 47, 89, 120; drug trafficking and, 102, 103; expatriates from, 30, 47, 65, 90, 95, 101, 104, 105
Franco-Prussian War, 22–23
French Assembly, 21

French Equatorial Africa, 23. *See also* Cameroon; Chad; Congo; Gabon
French Parliament, 35
French West Africa. *See* Afrique occidentale française (AOF)
French-Algerian War, 34

Gabon, 46, 106, 116
Gambia, 98, 108–109, 114
Gao, 29, 36
Garcin, Dr., 26, 101
Garvey, Marcus, 46
Gaye, François, 59, 66, 140n41
Gaye, Thérèze Diop, 59
gender, 3, 5, 12, 40, 42, 54, 59, 60, 62, 64, 65, 76, 77, 78, 95, 123
General Agreement on Tariffs and Trade (GATT) of 1994, 88
girls, 23–24, 28–29, 32, 33, 37
Girls' Preparatory School, 28–29
Gorée Island, 7, 8, 18, 23, 32
Grand Dakar, 69, 92
Guéye, Marie, 63
Guéye, Rokhaya Sylla, 94
Guigon, Bernard, 43, 63
Guigon, Henri, 27–28, 42

health and sickness, 2, 6, 13, 14, 17, 40–41, 81, 98, 111, 125
health care professionals. *See* medical professionals
Hibou, Beatrice, 97, 99
hospitals: colonial, 8, 17, 18, 20, 21, 22, 26, 28, 29, 31, 49; postcolonial, 83, 86, 95, 108, 109, 113, 115, 116, 118; Western European, 15, 18
Houillon, Frédéric, 29
Houphouët-Boigny, Félix, 29–30, 46

illegal pharmaceutical trade, 44, 97, 98–105, 116–17, 119, 121

Donna A. Patterson is Assistant Professor of Africana Studies at Wellesley College.